Warrior:
Built To Last

by Nacole Ali

Table of Contents

Nacole Ali

ACKNOWLEDGEMENTS

I want to personally thank the following people for their contributions to my inspiration in creating this book. My mother Jacqueline and Step-father Everett for all of your love, encouragement and prayers even though you are fighting your own battles; we will beat this! Thank you to my support team, my ace Meisha C. Holmes for all that you have done for me since day one, I can never repay you, Rochelle-Rona Magno for offering me the most precious thing a woman could offer; your hair to make a wig and entrusting me with your house keys, Akindra Daniels for all of the meals you cooked and real talk conversation about what this illness is really about, I know I know leafy greens lol, my godmother Juanita Thaxton for all of your unconditional love and support and standing by my side and taking care of me, my cousins Ronee Mattingly, Chemeine Mattingly, Dr. Katrina Mattingly, Dr. Monique Mattingly, Mahlik Richard aka Nino Khayyam, and Vernessa Richard, for the constant support, my niece Katherine for your gifts and love, my nephew Ryan for all your support, my niece Amber, my uncles Fred and Gary for always checking on me, my cousin Joe for running to the store for me, baby Sonja for giving me joy during recovery, my god-brother Kevin S. Parker for being there whenever needed and helping me through my new normal, my friend for decades Big Bub for listening and for gifting me with his amazing talent and voice and creating Dreamer – what an amazing song, my friend for over 30 years Chad Elliott, my college roomies, Deeyah and Tsahi for always holding me down. My brothers Mr. Walt and Evil Dee aka Da Beatminzers thank you for always thinking of me and loving me unconditionally. My brother Toby thank you for always making me laugh. The Nic to my Nac – Nicole thank you for listening. And to Natalie, Teon, Danny, and Diana thanks for all your support. Monica you are always showing up and showing out even when I don't expect it. EZ and Dr. Brian McNeil thank you much for your continued support. Kharisima thank you for your prayers, notes and care packages. And to all of my family and friends for your support from a far with your prayers, cards, emails, flowers, jokes, books, and conversation to get me through; I love you all.

To my amazing dream team at MSKCC. Thank you, thank you, thank you for helping me to continue to live my life with hope. Through all of my ups and downs Dr. Balsalga you have truly been a God send. To my surgeons, my nurses, my chemotherapy nurses, my awesome radiation team, and all of the assistants you all have made this process much easier than I ever expected even when I didn't want to listen.

And let me not forget the ones who disappeared during my process. You will never be forgotten, and thank you for showing me your true self.

DEDICATION

I dedicate this book to all my loved ones that have lost their battle with cancer, those that are still fighting and those that are survivors. Thank you for your unconditional love and encouragement.

JAT, LSM, GEM, CA, BT, RNT, DR.

I also dedicate this book to

my grandmother Dr. Vera D. Mattingly

for instilling in me the value of education and encouraging me to always do my best.

I love you.

Sunrise Sept. 1923 – Sunset Aug. 2013

WHO AM I
FOREWORD OF ME

I am a Brooklyn girl at heart. With that said, my character is filled with strength, determination, and fearlessness. I am a Christian, Corporate America working, college educated, entrepreneur, world traveler, funny (so I think), loving family and friends, spiritual, single, no children, and never married. Did I mention never married? Okay, moving on....

I am me. I do not desire to be any one but me. I do not let degrees, and jobs define me; they help mold me. I believe in helping those that want to help themselves. I believe in exploring other options (in most categories of my life). I don't stop at the first no. I don't like being taking advantage of. I believe in me first, but I am not selfish. I like pretty things. I like the finer things in life, but it doesn't mean I over extend myself to get it. I like being organized. I love to laugh. I love good food. I like being me, and I am always working on a better version. This is who I am. I am a beautiful woman of color.

"When life gives me lemons, I make pink lemonade" – Nacole Ali

Disclaimer:
Please pardon any errors since I texted this whole book. lol

INTRODUCTION

There is nothing worse than being diagnosed with a critical illness. I was diagnosed with stage 2 Breast Cancer. Within the week, my copays were up to $2000, and some of my medications that I need every other week had a $300 co-pay alone.

Besides the unexpected financial burden, there is a mental component to surviving this illness and regardless of the support team that may be around, it is ultimately up to the person to want to survive. It is hard to ask for help, it is hard to focus, and it is hard to comprehend all that is happening at the time it is happening.

I want to help create awareness so that more women get examined, and do not choose death over life because of the expenses associated with this disease or family obligations. I want to help save lives.

If women do not go for regular mammograms, there may be an increased chance of being diagnosed with more advanced breast cancers. Also, according to documented research, access to follow-up care after an abnormal mammogram may also contribute to the death rate.

It is a known fact that women who are diagnosed with later stage breast cancers have less chance of survival. For women in the U.S., breast cancer death rates are higher than those for any other cancer, besides lung cancer.

Gentlemen, this is not just a woman's disease. About 2,600 new cases of invasive breast cancer are expected to be diagnosed in men in 2016. A man's lifetime risk of breast cancer is about 1 in 1,000. 2013 there were an estimated 27,060 new cases and 6,080 deaths.

You cannot help anyone else if you are not healthy. Take action and schedule your mammogram appointment today.

1

Feb I Worry

Waiting To Exhale

Beep, beep, beep, beep awakened by the dreadful noise of a NYC garbage truck backing up. Monday morning 6:00am, peeking with one eye through the window of my boyfriend's studio apartment in Brooklyn; it's still dark. With short sluggish shuffles, scratching one butt cheek, I headed to the bathroom for a shower. I knew I had to get moving or I would be subjected to an over-crowded, stinky Manhattan bound 2 train; which I so despised. My eyes refocused and adjusted to the bright lights, as my feet were slowly moving towards the bathtub. Perfectly arranging the shower water between hot and lukewarm water, I quickly submerged under the heavy force of the shower. My entire body relaxed instantly. Ahhhh, relate, relax, and release; I exhaled. Lathering up, the bathroom was filled with a heavenly vanilla aroma. I was at ease. With suds scaling down my body, I ran my right hand across my left breast. Whoop, what was that? That ain't right, I thought to myself. (*Yes, I am college educated but I sometimes speak broken English in my head – keep reading – geesh*)

The nipple on my left breast was not as perky as it would normally be during a shower. My nerves were unsteady a bit but not exactly freaking out. I stepped out of the shower and looked into the mirror that reflected a curvaceous figure of a brown skin with long dark hair, and what seems to be an inverted nipple. (*Ok so I have a few more curves than what I use to have – lol*) When I looked down, my nipple literally looked partially dented inward. This was the first time I ever noticed this. Now staring at it, I didn't see any swelling marks, no itchy feel or discomfort; just awkwardness with my own body. I grabbed my cellphone off the sink and started taking pictures. (*Yes, my cell phone goes everywhere with me, most of the time, stop judging. Doesn't everyone take their cell phone into the bathroom with them?*) Anyway, I wanted to get a better look from a different angle and I wanted to compare photos in a few days to make sure it was getting better not worse. Finally feeling compelled to know more about my body's oddity, after toweling off, I Googled it. (*That is what I do people, I am a Google queen. After all Google, is my primary doctor and therapist Lol! Isn't it yours?*) I was just going to have to be late getting into the office. Dr. G. had over 139,000,000 results come up. And of course I go straight to the images. All sorts of images displayed different breast sizes and shapes, body disfigurements; Gross! However, most pictures and articles were leading to one thing.

I looked up at the time on the cable box, shit I was late for work. With my health heavy on my mind, my crappy commute was non-existent. As soon as I arrived in the office, I made a doctor's appointment with my real general practitioner, for my annual physical. I was lucky enough that by Friday, I visited my doctor, had blood work done, and asked for a referral for a mammogram. I was able to get a mammogram for the following Tuesday. My results showed my blood work was fine, which didn't indicate anything was wrong at that time. But my inner self was definitely saying something different. During the mammogram I was asked to take off everything from the waist up. The technician gave me what felt like a metal waist apron to put on for protection of my lower body from radiation. I stepped in front of the machine and placed my left breast on the cold flat surface. (*Okay, so yes I belong to the itty bity committee, what was I placing where?*) The technician repositioned my breast to get the exact correct angle. The technician told me to stand still and take

22

a deep breath. I watched a clear, plastic, square-shaped box lower and squeeze my itty bitty breast flat down to the height of a pancake. When the technician felt she had my breast clamped in well enough, she dashed off to snap an image on the computer. Once the image was successfully taken, she released the pressure of the machine and I exhaled. It was uncomfortable but quick, and thank goodness – ouch!   The process was done a few times on each breast at different angles.

"What do you see?" I asked. The technician told me, "You will have to wait for the doctor to discuss your results." With my right eyebrow up towards the ceiling, I didn't ask any more questions. After the mammogram, the technician instructed me to have a seat. She excused herself and within a few minutes she came back and asked if I could wait about an hour as I would need a sonogram. I agreed. The time crept slowly as I kept looking at clock on the wall. (*There is an old saying that says a watch clock does not tick. I get it now.*)

The technician came back and ask that I follow her into another exam room. She asked me to lay on the bed as she proceeded to squeeze a cold gel on my left breast. She used a small probe with a roller on the end to move all around the breast applying uncomfortable pressure so she could take more internal pictures. While she was scrolling back and forth across my breast, my intuition was tapping on my conscious giving me an unsettling feeling. I had a feeling they saw something abnormal. The focus was on my left breast, and once the exam was over, the cold gel was wiped off and I was asked to get dressed, and wait for the doctor. I started to get a little worried as the process went on a little further than expected. Impatiently waiting, flipping through the pages of fashion magazines in the waiting room, watching other woman come and go.

I kept telling myself, "This is not what I think it is; all this silly fuss over a funny-looking nipple?" (*Right! I was optimistically in denial*) The sonogram captured a different depth of images and helped the doctor to detect sizing of any abnormal masses. My results from the sonogram led the doctor to asking me to schedule another appointment two days later--but this time for a biopsy. My right eyebrow was sure getting a lot of exercise.

The doctor said, "The biopsy will determine if the suspicious mass is malignant or benign." I looked at her and nodded that I understood and I made an appointment near my office.

Thursday is here and when I arrived, it was evident that I was the youngest woman in the waiting area. Another obvious observation was that I was the only woman of color. What made me feel uneasy and the worst was walking in and thinking that everyone in the room knew about my condition, my secret. It was in their eyes; it was crazy that they all seem to have a look of concern for me or something; they knew why I was there. My inner thoughts are messing with me. Maybe it was written on my face? Paranoia had officially set in. I had to relax and just calm down but who the hell could be calm in this moment, in this environment? My mind raced with thoughts, all of the things I had been reading on Dr. G's web results including 200,000 new cases of Breast Cancer per year. Thinking to myself, I am a fairly healthy woman, I eat right for the most part, I exercise occasionally, never drank, and I surely never smoked. This is all probably for nothing. I have dense cystic breast and this is just precautionary, I thought to myself. These thoughts helped ease my mind a little, just a little. Why would I be sick? I assumed they were all ill and I was fine. I was lost in my own thoughts and by the time I looked up from my daze, the nurse had called my name several times. Feeling a bit spaced out, I stood and followed her while praying it was not that serious. This was the beginning of my denial stage. I walked away with the nurse looking back in slow motion at the others in the waiting room like I would never see them again.

(Queue the theme music of an old horror film. Queue the dim lights. Queue the sound of squeaky doors. Everyone quite on the set.)

It was almost like one of those movies where the hallway never ends, the corridors seemed to have stretched further, and further elongating as we walked. Maybe my mind was playing tricks on me. For a moment, I thought I was in Nightmare on Elm Street and Freddy was right behind me. The creepiest part was after we entered another waiting room with lockers, I was asked to undress from the waist up and was given the clinic's overused cotton blend polyester robe to put on. *(Don't judge, I was hoping for a terry cloth plush robe like at the spa.)* "Please have the opening to the front" the nurse said. Thinking to myself, is it possible the women were here for the exact same reason I was? As I sat down nervously thumbing through magazines, with my right leg shaking uncontrollably, I had an unnerving feeling. My anxiety was at a level 10. "Nacole Ali, Nacole Ali" the nurse called, it was my turn to go in the biopsy room. Standing up slowly, and living in slow motion for the first few seconds while I followed the nurse, I glanced at those sitting waiting their turn to be seen. (*Queue in How Do I Say Goodbye the theme song for Cooley High – yes I was feeling dramatic. I see some of you will need to have access to YouTube while reading so you can get the full effect of my emotional state*)

The nurse gave me a series of instructions then I settled myself on the table making sure I had my prayer cards in my back pocket, my cross in my front jean pocket, and I asked Jesus to take the wheel. I lifted my left arm above my head as instructed. The doctor explained what would happen next.

As I turned my head away from her, the doctor administered local anesthesia to numb an area of my breast. "It will be painless" the doctor said, just a small 1/10th of an incision. Then the doctor went into the incision with a little wand with

28

clamps on both ends to pull out pieces of tissue. She asked me if I felt anything, I replied "No." "Don't jump, please stay still as possible. Okay?" the doctor was confirming with me. "You are going to hear a weird sound." My mouth said okay, but in my R. Kelly voice my mind was telling me no. "Ok like wait, no, ok, no, wait, Lord Almighty" I said inhaling. The doctor re-entered again and the sound was like a construction worker's staple gun, Ga-gush! The doctor marked the lumpy area on the inside of breast with a titanium sort of clamp. The mechanical sound that resonated throughout the room would have made anyone uncomfortable. It scared the bejesus out of me. *(Is bejesus a word? Okay it is I just looked it up)* "Can you feel that?" asked the doctor. Was she joking? "Yes, of course I felt the clamp" I belted with attitude from pain. A second area on the same breast was numbed with more anesthesia as the doctor was making the incision. "How about now? Can you feel that?" said the doctor. Almost pleading I replied "Yes, all of it" as I was squeezing the hand of the nurse. Was she testing my patience? I thought to myself. Sore and depleted, I could feel every bit of the probe digging for clues, as if her name were Sherlock. She told me the procedure had to continue and how she was entering close to my nipple. I was in excruciating pain now, screaming at this point, looking straight up at the ceiling with tears rolling down the side of my face and into my ears. The local anesthesia was not working, I repeat, not working. The doctor was completely apologetic explaining that the area was very sensitive. With tears falling faster and faster to the sides of my face hitting the paper wrapped pillow I was laying on, I begged for her to hurry up and finish. My trembling body was immersed in fear, pain, sweat and confusion. This may sound crazy but for a moment it felt like I was in a S&M fetish movie with my nipple hoisted from the ceilings, back arched, and probes pulling from every angle--Oh the pain! (*Can you imagine? You can? Oh you kinky – lol.*) Finally, she got the sample she needed and it was over. The traumatic ordeal was finally over. Surprisingly, this procedure took about an hour in total though it felt like eternity. The samples would be sent off to the pathologists for examination and I was left feeling hurt and confused.

The doctor came back into the room once I was dressed. "Well, you know this isn't the worst case of cancer you could have" she said. Say what now? My lip started to quiver. Did she diagnosed me without even getting the results? My face froze and tears fell. All of what she said seemed to have come out in slow motion. I stopped listening and was caught up in my thoughts, I clinched the cross in my pocket and started to scream at the top of my lungs, letting out a dreadful howl. I thought to myself, "I'm going to die." The nurse tried to console me for a bit then gave me a few minutes alone to process the news as she walked out.

About twenty minutes later, I got myself together, collected my things and left. I wiped my tears and continued my day as normal, trying hard not to think about the diagnosis. From the appointment, I went back to work as if nothing happened.

The following day, I attended a birthday gathering for my good friend Raquel. After work I went directly to a cousin's house to pick her up so we could drive together. During the drive to New Jersey, it didn't take long for Michele to figure out that something was wrong that night because I was stand-offish. I had nothing to tell really, the actual results from the tests would come in a few days. The mass could be benign and everything would be fine. Though my spirit was down and my breast was sore, I pushed myself through the rest of the day trying to avoid what I was feeling. We arrived at the dine-in theater where Raquel was having her birthday gathering. We ordered food. "Are you alright?" Michele consistently asked. "Yeah, I'm fine." Lying through my teeth. "Whatever, you will tell me when you want to tell me" she said, and it was left at that. *(Lights out - movie started)*

The drive home was a little awkward. The entire ride I was contemplating, what to say, and how to say it. We pulled up to Michele's mother's house in Brooklyn where she parked her car and I blurted out "I had a biopsy yesterday and there is a possibility that I have breast cancer." Surprisingly, her reaction was upbeat and supportive. Michele talked about what we should do and if I needed anything she would be available. I appreciated her understanding and it meant a lot to hear her say these words. I needed to talk about it with someone because it was making me crazy with worry. I drove off and headed to my boyfriend's house. I called my godmother to inform her of the same, as a nurse, her response was soooooo different. She was the reality check I was not looking for. "Well you know you are in denial" she said. "Just get prepared and let me know what the doctor says, I am here if you need me." "Ok, have a good night" she said.

Trying to not let her words resonate, I disconnected the call, and it was late so I kept it short. I arrived at my boyfriend's house and headed straight to bed without a peep. The stress of the day had me wore down like a heel on an old pair of shoes and the soreness of the biopsy from the day before had me shattered. Saturday morning Michele called to see how I was feeling, and explained how she had a hysterical breakdown for about twenty minutes in the street once I drove off. My heart sank after I heard this. I decided that I would not tell anyone else until I knew for sure.

I stayed at my boyfriend's house about a week or so until maintenance work was completed at my place. First thing Monday morning I started to call the doctor's office, the suspense of waiting for the doctor to call was killing me. It felt like eternity waiting for my official prognosis. I called and called and waited.

By late afternoon, I finally got through to the doctor's office. "Hi, Nacole. Are you alone?" I plopped down on the sofa with heaviness in my stomach. No one ever calls asking if you are alone

34

if they are about to give you a good news. I knew the worst part was coming. "Yes, I am. What are my results?" She said, "Nacole, you have breast cancer."

A ton of bricks fell in the middle of my chest, it was hard to breath. It was finally confirmed. The voice on the phone went on to instruct me in making appointments with doctors and surgeons. "How will I know what to do?" I asked. "You will find out more information from each specialist after each visit. They will tell you what to do" she replied. She gave me a referral for a surgeon. My ears heard everything she said but my mind was not totally convinced. In denial, I was still on the fence but listening to her advice as I went to Google searching for doctors. Through my research I found the top breast cancer centers in the nation. A well-known center was located in NYC. The next thing I had to do was find out if the hospital would accept my insurance since they had a slim list of providers. Thankfully the center accepted my current insurance plan. Next, I searched their website to look for doctors and made my appointments. My mind was focused and I went through the motions to make myself productive. My emotions were pushed aside for the moment. "Hi, I'm calling to make an appointment for the breast surgeon. I have been diagnosed with breast cancer. What's your next availability? Anything in the next two weeks?" I am not sure how often callers are cheerful when making appointments for cancer treatments but my mood seemed to have carried through the phone and to the receiver of the calls. One receptionist replied, "Well looks like you're in luck. We have an opening this Tuesday morning at 10 am." Was I hearing her right? I can have my checkup with one of the leading doctors in the nation within a day? "Wow, that's perfect! I will take it." I organized my schedule for the rest of the day, my paperwork, and planned out what I needed to do for the upcoming appointment. I was going to make sure all test results were available as requested by the hospital. Maybe it was the stress of feeling overwhelmed but the day went by in a flash with all that planning.

Tuesday morning arrived and I was anxious. The surgeon went over my test results and made her own suggestions. "We received your pathology report but we need to conduct our own tests." I know she did not just say I would have to go through another painful biopsy. Channeling my alter ego, Esto es una mierda or plainly speaking, 'This sucks!' *(I don't even speak Spanish, but thought it would be cool to say it in a different language and yes I double check with my primary Dr. G. he also translates - lol)* I wanted to slump in my chair and start kicking and screaming like a 2-year old, but I remained calm. "Excuse me? Will I have to be probed again, is that what you mean? That was quite painful the first time" I stated. I needed assurance the same nipple test would not be performed again in such a painful way. "Oh, no Nacole, don't worry. We will use the same tissue from your last biopsy" the surgeon said. With a sigh of relief, a sense of calm came over my body.

"When shall we schedule your surgery?" the doctor stated with sternness in her voice. "Wait what? Before we jump to surgery what are my options?" "Well we can try and shrink the tumor to preserve your breast and do a lumpectomy but right now based on the size I recommend a mastectomy" the doctor said plainly. "How can I preserve my breast?" I curiously said. "You would have to make an appointment with the oncologist" the doctor simply stated "Okay, I will do that" I said in a quiet tone.

I purposely asked the receptionist who is the best specialist in the field to take care of my case. The receptionist said oh that would be Dr. Bedoya, but it is almost impossible to get an appointment with him. I asked her to please look. She said "Oh you're in luck, I found an open slot for tomorrow afternoon with Dr. Bedoya." I couldn't believe it, my next visit was at the hospital with the leading oncologist specializing in breast cancer. I asked my boyfriend to drive me as he just so happened to have that Wednesday off.

(Queue the theme music, Feeling Good by Nina Simone. "It's a new dawn, it's a new day, it's a new life for me, and I am feeling good.")

Dr. Bedoya was a warm-hearted Spaniard with a sense of humor that helped me calm down tremendously. He was very straightforward with me and I appreciated that. He explained my condition thoroughly. "Look, you have to have chemotherapy Nacole. Now, there is a matter of surgery or chemotherapy first, but in the end, you will have to undergo chemotherapy either way." Even though I heard him loud and clear, I didn't seem to mind his instructions or perhaps it did not register at the time what those phrases exactly meant.

"You will have 16 sessions of chemotherapy scheduling one week on, one week off for now. The first 4 sessions of Adriamycin and

Cytoxan or A/C as they call it, which will be the harshest and taxing on your body. It's a combination of drugs supporting different functions in your system to attack the bad cells harming your body. Expect to be nauseated and fatigued after each visit for about 6-8 days. Additionally, there are some expected side effects, like skin discoloration and hair loss to name a few. Since you are premenopausal, you may or may not have a menstruation because of the chemotherapy. The decision is yours. Do you have any questions?" Dr. Bedoya said in a soft tone. "I have a scheduled trip to Italy on April 3rd. How can we make this chemo thing happen so I make the trip?" I didn't mind what the doctor was saying. I don't want my chemotherapy to be the reason why I won't be able to go. I didn't want the cancer to control my life. The doctor kind of chuckled and calmly explained, "In order for the chemotherapy to fully work, there needs to be a routine in place. You can't miss any doses. For the process to work best, you need consistency. But I do recommend if you are going

40

to start with chemotherapy we should start right away; starting next week."

Before we could discuss it any further he asked that I retrieve the pathology results from Mt. Sinai Hospital uptown before 5pm to begin the paperwork process. Just then something changed, motivation swept over me, and an unbelievable amount of energy. I felt like a warrior. (*Queue in Rocky theme music – Eye of the Tiger. Oh stop it you know you like the theme music references.*)

The way in which I was accepting my fate and taking on this lofty journey so quickly was mind boggling, I impressed myself. Right at that moment I decided to challenge myself further and get everything I needed for my chemotherapy to start next week. The pathology report from Mt. Sinai was the only way to get approved for chemotherapy so soon. I looked at my watch, it was already 3pm. I dashed out the door like my name was Flo Jo and jumped in the car with my cousin Randi and my boyfriend who was waiting downstairs for me. Talking fast telling him where to go, we raced uptown on 3rd Ave in the rain to get to the hospital. While my boyfriend dipped between taxis and buses, I was on the phone with Mt. Sinai to advise them I was in route, and to please have my results ready for pickup. Once I arrived at the hospital, I jumped out of the car and raced through to the security desk, my next challenge was to find out how to get to the 15th floor. "Where you wanna go?" the security guard appeared puzzled by my eagerness. I quickly looked for the paper in my bag where I wrote the information on and showed it to security. With perplexity and sounding like Foghorn Leghorn from Bugs Bunny, he said, "Hmmm... I don't know where this is. Ahhhh, wait here let me call my supervisor." He turned his back a walked like he had led in the heel of his shoes. Is this real? I thought to myself, am I being punk'd? Is Ashton Kutcher about to jump out and surprise me? I looked at my watch and it was now 3:50pm. Heart pumping and the sweat from my anxiety was making my face glisten like I just completed a 3 hour zumba class. *(I have never taken a 3 hour zumba class, this is just a visual for added drama)* The security guard walked slowly towards me, and in his country voice said pointing towards the door "What you wanna do is go back out this door, make a left, walk about two blocks and go to building 1000 on your left side." OMG! I turned around before he could finish; yelling thanks, ran out the door and slid over the hood of the car like I was in a Die Hard action movie and jumped back in the car. I told my boyfriend with anxiety to go up two more blocks and double park on the left side of the street. "What are you waiting for?" I screamed. He looked at me in slow motion and then looked up and said "It's a red light" "Oh!" I said calmly as if I already knew that. When the light turned green, he drove the two blocks and pulled up. I quickly ran in the building and went to security to find out where I needed to go. The security guard pointed me to the elevator bank on the opposite side of the lobby. I made a dash for the elevators as it was turning 4:10pm. I was out of breath and gasping for air but

I could not stop pressing the elevator button repeatedly. Finally, I arrived at the 15th floor of the correct building, and ran down the hallway to the records room. With shortness of breath I muttered, "Hi, I am here to pick up test results. I called earlier. My name is Nacole Ali." The receptionist found my results. "Okay here they are, that will be $120 dollars for your lab results mam." For the life of me I couldn't understand why I would have to pay out of pocket for lab results. Thinking quickly, I tried reasoning with the receptionist. "Excuse me, but how do lab results get to the doctors at the hospital?" I said with perplexity. "Oh, we usually bill the office directly" the clerk confirmed. "Well, let's pretend I'm a messenger service that needs to get the results to the doctor by 5pm; bill them directly please. Can you do that?" Sensing my urgency, she went with my suggestion and billed them directly. Who knew it could be so easy to persuade her. The amount of money was fine but the unexpectedness of paying sounded a bit off to me and I was in a rush. Everything was still so new

44

to me, and there was no way of predicting what would come next whether financially or physically.

I was hoping the traffic would be light on the way back to the hospital. Once the pathology reports were in my possession I ran back to the car, my boyfriend dipped and weaved through traffic like we were Bonnie and Clyde reaching the hospital by 4:55pm. OMG, my heart was pumping out of my chest. I exhaled. *(It's funny now, but back then, I think I lost 5 pounds and a lung.)* Most people probably aren't in a hurry to lose their hair and skin pigmentation, but like my grandmother always told me, I was a special girl.

I was determined to get this process started. At the moment I felt fine. I had lots of energy to do things. So I started being proactive in my breast cancer journey. From creating lists, to finding useful medical apps for my phone *(they actually exist)*, researching more information about different stages and chemo, I did it all. Officially, I was embracing the fact of life. I had breast cancer.

45

My mental approach to the situation was simple: since doctors said I have this thing, well I'm gonna fix it, easy as that. Or that's how I saw it. Realization and acceptance started seeping in day by day as denial slowly crept far away. For the first time since my awkward moment in the shower, I felt at ease and not so on edge anymore. My mind became a bit clear when I realized I had to let my job know about my condition. In addition, I wanted to tell my mother along with a few close family members. However, after my Cousin Michele's reaction, I would need to prepare myself to be stronger for them. It was evident that I had two choices. I could either lie down and cry about my condition or take the choice to do something about what fate had handed me, accept my new normal. And that is what it was, a situation that I chose to be positive about. Determined not to take on a victim role, I was going to do everything in my power to learn and understand the daunting task of curing myself of cancer. I never gave myself the time to have an anxiety attack about the start of this journey. In actuality, I never had much time to sulk at all. On some days my emotions would get the best of me but for the most part, at the moment, I could easily say I was okay.

A week full of doctor's appointments, testing and bad news had past and I figured it's near the weekend and I would tell my boyfriend on Saturday all that has happened. At this point he knew he was helping me gather documents, but not that I was officially diagnosed. I felt I should share the news with him as well since we had been dating for a year and a half and we had known each other for almost 25 years. He had been so supportive during the sunset of my grandmother and I knew he could emotionally support me when needed.

I woke up Saturday morning, and I headed to the kitchen to make something to eat; not far, he lives in a studio apartment remember. Soon the aroma of bacon and eggs woke him up. We sat at the coffee table eating breakfast. We sat for about ten minutes before I broke the news. "So what's on your mind? What did the doctor say?" His beautiful smile subsided to a face of discontentment as the words "I have breast cancer" uttered softly from my lips. He looked at me and used compassionate phrases like 'I am here for you' and 'we will get through this together'. He started asking me all of these questions, I did not have the answer to. (*What a cry baby I am turning into*) But the conversation started to shift, I don't even remember how, but in a split second, all of a sudden, the same man told me 'I am not prepared for this', 'I can't see you sick', and 'I don't think I can be here for you'. WTF? This bastard was breaking up with me now? After I shared the worst news of my life? I kept thinking what kind of person walks away when you need them the most? I began to cry from the anger and disappointment but my pride would not let me falter. Moments later I thanked him for his honesty and proceeded to violently pack my things. (*Rewind: I was furious and cursing him out, throwing stuff around, and having an out of body experience – now to back to our regularly scheduled program.)* I called Michele and told her what had just happened and asked her if I could stay with her. I finished packing my things and left. I never looked back and he never stopped me from walking away.

Refusing to continue to cry, my eyes were staring to look like strawberries – big and red. I immediately called Michele back from the car and told her the details. I could barely get the words out from anger. "Can you believe this asshole? I have so much on my mind and now this shit? I can't believe he's doing this to me!" I don't think I let her get a word in. What was happening? But, I had no time to sulk. I drove to Michele's house in a daze. I felt like every song on the radio was a sappy love song, and every advertisement was for a cancer center. Funny how whatever problems you have, seems all things on the television and radio relates to you and your situation. Once I reached my cousin's house, she sympathetically listened at first, and then became equally as perturbed as I was. We

Warrior Built To Last

fed off of each other's anger about the situation. We were knee deep in royally roasting my now ex-boyfriend when my Godmother called. Bringing the emotion down a notch, I had to tell her what happened from the doctor's visit. She was very calm and focused about what I should do. I must rename her RC (Reality Check) for many reasons. Funny enough, after I told her the news about my now x-boyfriend, she did not respond as I expected. She shared with me that it was better he left the relationship early on, versus waiting until things became worse. She said it would be worst emotionally if he waited and walked out on me while I were helpless, and weak. I guess she was right, but I still could not wrap my head around the situation. She calmed me down completely, and helped me focus the attention on me and helped to keep me positive throughout the day. I didn't need his stress right now. I needed time to try and understand what all was happening to me and what steps needed to be taken if any.

I stayed with Michele for the week and used my spare time to proactively research breast cancer on Dr. G and what it all meant. Looking back, this was probably the wrong thing to do. Even though I knew I had Breast Cancer, I started to try and figure out how I got it, checking for other abnormalities, and claiming symptoms I didn't have. One thing Google has perfected is providing an overkill of crap on the internet for people to believe, whether it be real or make-believe. But I needed to do something to keep my mind off of the doctor's results and the fact that I was once again single.

Unofficially diagnosed in January, but by the middle of February I was facing new challenges like a warrior. Through my never-ending research, constant question asking, and keeping track of doctor's appointments and now starting chemotherapy. When I informed my job about what happened, they of course were very sympathetic with me. They were happy to help in any way they could. I would need to take off days for appointments but I wanted to continue working. I believed that working would help keep my mental state healthy.

I gradually started to understand more about the diagnosis and what everything meant in accord with my daily pattern of life. With this new confidence, I knew what I had to do next. I had to deal with the emotional burden and courage of telling key members in my family. Telling my mom was going to be tough. I hadn't even mentioned it to her at this point for a good reason. Growing up, I saw my mom battle through several health issues and I didn't want to burden her spirits with the news, as she was in her own battle with lung cancer, but it had to be done.

Starting with telling the rest of my family, I felt it necessary to tell my niece. It was hard but I felt she should know what was going on. I told my female cousins first. I thought about how my diagnosis could affect others around me as well. My cousins who are around the same age as me who could possibly be at risk. Instead of telling each cousin one by one, I set up a conference call for the upcoming weekend to inform them of the news.

Some of my family members took the news well, others didn't. Understandably so, I realized not everyone is good at handling bad news or might immediately think of death when cancer is mentioned. But I kept bright and upbeat as I revealed all the information from the doctors. One cousin in particular had to be consoled which was funny since I was the sick one. *(Okay, this is what kills me about telling people about my condition, I end up having to console them, I end up having to ensure them that I am going to be all right – not for nothing but what part of the game is this. Just venting.)* I also noticed that I had to separate myself from over sympathetic or over emotional reactions because it brought my spirit down. I wanted to keep the positive energy that I cultivated because I knew it would help to get me through it all. In the end, their responses were pretty positive:

"Whatever you need, let us know."

"Call me. Don't hesitate if you need something."

"I'll call and check on you to make sure you're okay." Not for nothing but for the most part when people say those things, it's – a statement. They are never truly in it for the long haul. So take it with a grain of salt, because out 9 of 10 of them are full of shit....

The social worker at the hospital warned me. She said I will lose friends and I will gain friends. I didn't know what she meant at the time, but I know now. However, I felt the needed to separate myself from some people at times to not only save them from internalizing my illness, but to have time for multitasking appointments and giving a fair amount of quality time to myself for healing and not being bombarded with questions.

On my journey to start chemotherapy, I made arrangements with my godmother and my cousin Michele to stay in Brooklyn, so I could have easy access to the hospital. For the first time in my life I was asking for help. Truly this is a new day. *(Y'all don't even know my struggle)*

I woke up on the chilly Tuesday morning of February 17th it was a normal day for everyone else. For me, it was my first chemotherapy treatment. My cousin took me to my first appointment and I admit I had no particular emotion that day. In fact, I felt fine. Still, at this point, there weren't any visible signs or health complications. When I arrived at the hospital, they took my vitals, I saw my oncologist, and then I was escorted to a small private room with a comfortable chair and machines with several IV bags.

I sat and eased into the chair to prepare myself for a long time of sitting. The hospital told me to expect to stay about 5 - 6 hours in most cases. The friendly nurse who escorted me to the treatment room explained what would happen that day. She checked my vitals again to make sure I was prepared for treatment. Everything was a go for chemotherapy. Waiting patiently, over an hour later my custom-made cocktail ordered by my physician and prepared by the pharmacist was ready. They always tell you 'Some side effects may occur'. It just depends on the drug being used and how your body will respond to treatment. The fine print - Some people experience nausea, vomiting, hair loss, mouth sores, diarrhea, rashes, and/or fatigue. Are they kidding? My optimistic behind thought well, I will just do everything in my power to avoid this side effects. But truth be told, this alone had me thinking. What is in this stuff? So here's the problem, chemotherapy kills good cells and the bad cells that were constantly dividing rapidly out of control in my system. That's the cause of the side effects. The medication destroys all cells *(All right information overload, but necessary.)*

Soon, the nurse began the procedure. The nurse looked at my arms and started searching for the perfect veins for the pre-meds, I could feel the fluid going through my body in the beginning but after a while the slight sting subsided. The medication made me sleepy and sluggish. I kept my body as relaxed as possible because I knew it would help things move along more smoothly. So relaxed, I was in a good sleep, with two heated blankets on. Plus I was not trying to focus on all the machines beeping, and people coming in and out of my room. Based on the type of cancer I have, my chemo treatment would take about 5 months in total. For the first 4 treatments, I took chemo orally for the following 2 days, separated with weekly breaks. This was all to help me fight this disease. Feeling a different range of emotions, I tried to just focus on what was happening at the moment. Medicine was entering my system through my veins to help me cure my illness. This is what I was sure of. As much as I may have had a support system, this is my personal journey that I will have to withstand to go through alone. The social worker was right, I feel alone.

My first chemo session was over and the nurse called a prescription into my pharmacy for a shot to keep up my white blood cell count. Michele and her boyfriend drove me to the pharmacy only to be told I had a $600 co pay. I could not believe my ears. Is that right? Are they serious? Is this another prank? $600 and I will need three more of these? Ok something has got to give. So I politely ask the pharmacist, to help me understand my options. He said the only thing we can do is, get special services on the phone, maybe they can assist you. Foot tapping, and eyebrow raised, I patiently waited, what's a couple of more minutes? Super annoyed. "This is special services; how can I assist you?" Already with frustration in my voice "Yes, I am here at the pharmacy and they told me that my prescription co-pay was $600." "That is correct" the voice replied. "I don't have $600 to give you, so what are my options?" I was put on hold, I felt like I was holding forever. The representative finally came back on the line to say there is nothing they can do. Well, that's when I hit the roof with steam coming out of my ears, like a cartoon character. By this time I had an audience at the pharmacy. *(I felt like Oprah in the color purple – "Oh Mrs. Sophia home now!")* I said in a stern voice through my teeth, rocking back and forth "You are not going to make the decision weather I live or die, I am choosing to live. But this is what I do know, I am walking out of here with my prescription. *(I saw a quick flash of the news: Woman runs out of pharmacy with medication – I can do this if I have too – Man who was I fooling, I have never stolen anything in my life – was this going to be the first - news at 11)* You don't have the right to make people choose between living and feeding their family." I am disgusted. I sounded like the exorcists. "Please hold" I heard the voice on the other end of the receiver say. What felt like 10 minutes of silence, not even hold music, the rep finally came back on the phone to say "We will bill you monthly for 6 months, if that is alright with you, can I please speak to the pharmacist?" I agreed and happily handed over the phone. The pharmacist then handed me a huge ice packed box. *(Did I mention when I was plotting to take my meds, they were behind the counter? Oh the drama)*

"What the hell took you so long?" Michele shouted from the front seat of the car "Drama with the pharmacy" I calmly explained. My body was drained and I wanted to just get home quickly to assess how my body would react to my first treatment. Once we got to Brooklyn we unpacked the huge box to find a little box inside that needed to be refrigerated. Every day was a new learning experience and this was a hard but useful lesson. I called my godmother as she agreed to give me a shot when it was time. She heard the exhaustion and stress in my voice. "You okay Nacole? What happened?" Not wanting to repeat the story again I just explained that I would tell her about it when I come over. She agreed and understood.

"You know what I just realized? This is about to be an expensive journey" I randomly said to my cousin. The realization of how financially taxing cancer treatment would be, hit me at that moment. I wondered how many people really understood what financial burden cancer recovery is, or how many people would have just walked out of the pharmacy all together. Unnecessary stress. Slept like a baby that first night though. Those drugs knocked me on my butt.

The next day, first thing when I woke up, I checked the pillow for lost hair, I didn't know what to expect. I waited for my godmother to get home, and went to get my shot. I felt okay but my energy was down. I felt like I had been working a double shift with no sleep. I gave her the box out of the packaging. She said okay smiling "I will inject you in your butt, you have enough you won't even feel it." Lord help me. Is this going to hurt? Will I be able to sit? I was thinking to myself "Well, let's get this over and done with" I said. Looking away. I didn't flinch as she stuck me. "We're done" she said. I pulled up my pants and laid down on the bed. I needed a rest.

Two days later I could hear the doctor's words echoed in my mind "6-7 days after your first treatment your hair might fall out." I was actually sitting around waiting for this event like waiting and watching for the groundhog to come up out of the ground to inform us about the end of winter.

2

March Forward

A Solider Story

(Damn for the shortest month of the year, February sure was a longgggg month, wasn't it?) I'm not feeling too bad after my first treatment. I went on about my days trying to get some work done at home. Most of my time was spent reading up on literature about cancer stages but specifically hair loss. I read that some people wait until it falls off chuck by chuck. Others would cut their hair in advance down to a low haircut. I was thinking I should be proactive, not sure I could watch my hair fall out in chunks and I could not see myself shaving my head bald either. I thought about it for a while then called my old friend Ed that owned a barber shop in Brooklyn. I spoke frankly with him about what I was planning to do. "Look, here's the

deal. I've been diagnosed with breast cancer and I want to cut my hair. Specifically, I want you to cut my hair, Ed. Will you do it?" We chatted for a while and he didn't pry at first but just listened as I explained why I needed to cut my hair. He was naturally supportive but his militant views about my treatment became immediately apparent. "Nacole, come on! You're not going on that chemo for real are you? You know what? That's big brother's poison. That's just the government wanting you to die slow using their prescription drugs that you have to pay for. They want you to pay for your own death. There are plenty of alternatives, you can eat better and take herbal supplements. Don't let the man tell you your only option in chemo!" Ed passionately responded. Oh boy, I should have known, but I stayed calm, and let him finish. He continued "Listen man, you can't take all those drugs Nacole. Are you eating right?" Rolling my eyes. "Don't worry Ed, I have my own formula. I am going to combine a mix of modern medicine and alternative methods. I plan on continuing my treatments but also I'm focusing on nutritional health and maintaining a healthy diet. This will help the drugs to do what they are supposed to do" I explained with a calm demeanor. "Listen sister, there are alternatives you know, Right?" "Yes, I am aware of alternatives Ed, but right now I just need you to cut my hair. Please? Can you do that, Malcom X?" He dropped the topic. "Okay, okay. So how you want to get it cut?"

"Well, I'm a little embarrassed."

"Why? Ladies come in and shave their heads all the time. It's normal."

"Well, I haven't had short hair since I was a young. You know as long as you've known me, it's never been short. I've always kept it medium to long lengths."

"No problem hun. No need to be embarrassed. Matter of fact, here's what we will do. I will open the shop for you only, so that you will have privacy. We can arrange it for a Sunday so that it doesn't affect business hours. You know what? I have an even better idea. You should tell some of your girls to come as well. You know what I mean? You know make it an event. Have them come and support you."

"Okay cool, I will see you Sunday."

Without hesitation, after hanging up with Ed, I called a few of my close friends that knew that I was diagnosed.

The upcoming Sunday afternoon my friends met up with me in Brooklyn at Ed's barber shop. They brought along their cheerful smiles and laughter which filled the room with lots of love and made me more at ease. When I pulled up front and saw my longtime friend Ed standing inside the shop, I felt glad he was helping me. As I stepped closer towards the shop he grabbed me with both arms and gave me the biggest bear hug to show no love was lost during that long time that we were apart. I introduced my friends to him and everyone was cordial. While my friends chatted amongst themselves I stared in the mirror at my hair for a long time. I ran my fingers through it and really noticed it for the first time. It's just hair, it can grow back, I thought to myself. I was ready for the change.

"Hey Nacole, YOU READY?" Ed shouted. Without a response, Ed asked me to sit. He snapped the apron around to the back of my neck. As, I sat in his barber chair still, I noticed every movement and sound behind me. My friends and Ed agreed on a nice short cut. I even showed him some pictures that I saw online that I thought would look good. Michele, April, Raquel, Randi, and Chris, had not said a word while everyone was listening to the sound of the clippers. "Lower your head" Ed directed. BUZZZZ…. I lowered my head and listened to the sound from the clippers. My hair was being cut an inch from my scalp! I squeezed tightly to the barber chair, bracing myself for the worse. I felt the first pass of the clippers through my hair. I felt fine. It wasn't so bad after all. I thought I'd get emotional or cry, since that had been my M O since I was diagnosed. None of that happened. Maybe it was the support of my friends, funny jokes and laughter that helped. I stared at the hair on the floor. Nothing. I was really okay. Soon it was all over. I looked at the new Nacole in the mirror. She looked so different from a few minutes ago. But in a way, this Nacole looked confident and not afraid to take on new challenges. Cutting my hair was symbolic to how I would face adversities during my journey. When a problem arises, accept it, roll with it and find the next solution, is my typical attitude, so why change now? It was truly a practice of acceptance, letting go, and courage. I never fully understood the extent of my strength until this moment. I thanked Ed for helping me by returning his bear hug with one of my own. We took a few pictures for memories of what went down that day. After we left the barbershop and said our goodbyes to Ed, my girls and I went out to grab something to eat at a nearby soul food restaurant.

Yess, honey, looking at myself in the mirror. It didn't take long for me to fall in love with my new hairdo. The change was liberating because I didn't have to do anything. I just loved waking up in the morning without pressing, curling, and blow drying my hair. Hmmm maybe chemo, not so bad, I started to notice some perks. I know some people would naturally think everything negative about going through treatment but I wanted to focus on some of the positives my body would go through.

Soon the hair on my body started to fall off in different places. Gradually, I didn't have hair under my arms or pubic area. Yes! Finally, a perk. As, I looked in the mirror and smirked. This isn't that bad. I started to realize some of the small beneficial events that were happening due to the treatment. Each morning I woke up and examined my body in the mirror wondering when more of my hair would disappear. "I don't have to shave!" thinking to myself after noticing nothing was there anymore. *(Okay so wait allllll my hair is gone – I don't even have hair in my nose – who knew?)*

The bathroom is a place a frequent visit as I always have to go. But I am starting to notice every time I pee, I now have to wash my inner thighs. I can't pee straight. What part of the game is this? The phone rang and it was Randi.

"Hey what's up gurly" she said with her chipper voice.

"Auhhh, I can't pee straight" I replied.

Hearing a bunch of noise on the phone "Wait what?"

"I can't pee straight" repeating myself.

Always asking me clarifying questions, Randi says "What do you mean exactly? Like you can't pee in the toilet?" "When I pee, it goes all over the place, I end up having to wash my butt and thighs after every pee" I clarified. After a hysterical laugh Randi says "Oh got it. Okay this is what you have to do - go to the pleasure chest in the city and buy a pee cup."

Sitting up straight in my chair "Where? To get what?" I said with confusion.

"It's called Go Girl. Google it" laughing hysterically she said. I was so confused, now I had questions. "You go to the Pleasure Chest?" "You have a pee cup?" "How do you know about these things?" "What do you need a pee cup for?" she quickly dodged the question. "Never mind. Get out of my business. Oh, look you can order it online!" *(Story in a nutshell, I ordered it and it worked, just not cool when you are not home. But it helped. And Randi are you really not going to tell me how you know about the pee cup?)*

During my next doctor visit, the nurse asked, "Are you currently having a cycle?" Smiling "No, not at the moment." Writing her notes "Well, good. You probably won't get a cycle during treatment and some women are even known not to get a cycle at all." "I'll take it" I said showing all my teeth. I can deal with that. My body must be adjusting well; I haven't been feeling so bad after all besides a little fatigue. (*Disclaimer, this is only the beginning.*)

I was looking for a bright spot in all of the darkness I was going through. After all, at the moment, I was lacking emotional support. Unfortunately, the initial people who said that they would be around for me if I needed anything slowly started to disappear. I was mainly alone, mentally and physically. I was learning a valuable lesson in life. I began to understand that only I can help myself. As a woman it is our natural instant to take care of others before ourselves, and I had done so for so many years, I had let my own well-being demise. What a lesson to learn at a time like this. This forced me to grow, learn myself, and challenge myself in areas that were foreign to me. I was going through a metamorphosis, a transformation. I will say that those I least expected to be present through my journey showed up to appointments and later hospital visits. At some point, I had to realize that this was my issue and not those of my loved ones. I have to force myself to do for me and to get up and go to appointments. I cannot expect others to reschedule their lives for me. So I accepted whatever help I could get and continued to do what was in my best interest. I had to learn how to ask for help. I stayed emotionally strong and pulled myself together and managed on my own. I tried to make myself to be as normal as possible when people asked me to go to different places, knowing I probably would get tired or wouldn't be able to finish a meal at a restaurant due to nausea or lack of appetite, I went anyway. Fake it 'til you make it, was the phrase that came to mind. There was no use in sulking and feeling bad for myself because it will just give me stress. I wanted to stay in a clear and positive mindset and so I did.

Two weeks later my second treatment was scheduled. I brought my iPad to surf the net for more research. *(Why? I now ask myself)*. The process was long as usual. I showed up on time but waited for about an hour before getting started with treatment. They took my vitals and reviewed my blood levels to see if I was all right for treatment. After the cocktail of medications were prepared for my treatment, I was taken to my private room to get comfortable for a long process.

I followed this session with my home administered shot to increase my white blood cell count. Then, oral chemotherapy pills for the next few days. This was my bi-weekly routine. I can't say I got used to any of it. I downloaded apps on my phone as reminders to take my meds. Raquel and I also started to document everything that was happening, play by play. Every visit felt a bit unique in a strange way. After my second treatment, I began to feel more physical changes. I felt very fatigued for the first time since treatment started. Like clockwork, the doctor was right about the side effects that would pop up the 6-8 days following chemotherapy. It started with little things like the shower would feel too hot though the temperature was lukewarm. I felt like I wanted to faint, but didn't recognize it right away as part of the side effects. There were moments of shortness of breath for no particular reason. The biggest proof came about when I took public transportation.

"Hey, Nacole you up?" Michele whispered through the crack in the door.

Looking at the door with one eye open "Yes" feeling groggy I slowly said.

Putting her head between the door frame and the door "I'm leaving at 7:30 if you want a ride to the train station." The train station was 5 blocks away and it was cold outside. "All right" I told her. But of course I looked at the clock and it was already 7:00am. I pulled myself together as fast as I could. I headed for the front door, and waited in the car with Michele's boyfriend. Bright and chipper "Good morning everyone" Michele said grinning from ear to ear, throwing her bags in the back seat of the car. "Come onnnnnn Michele" her boyfriend

76

said with his Caribbean accent. "You're gonna be late for work, let's go." As he rolled his eyes, and started the car. I sat in the back seat, watching these two like movie. A few minutes later, we are at the train station. On my way down the train station stairs, I already felt uneasy. It was like everyone knew what I was going through. My heart began to beat rapidly, and I began to sweat all of a sudden. The train was coming and everyone started to make a dash for their spot on the platform. I was feeling overly tired and hot. "Watch the closing doors please" the automated PA system recited, BING BONG. Crowds of people rushing and pushing into the train, with sounds of grunting, and teeth sucking. I pushed on to the train like everyone else. You would have thought this was the last train to get to heaven the way people desperately tried to fit. "People there is another train behind this one, if you do not fit, wait for the next train" the conductor yelled out the window of the train. I kept thinking to myself, I am so hot. The sweat started to bead on my forehead. I felt a tap on my shoulder. "Ms. Do you want to sit?" a calm voice behind me whispered. I shook my head yes, and a pathway opened up on the train like the parting of the Red Sea. At this point I figured I must be looking pretty bad, if someone on a crowed train gave up their seat, after all these are the same people that turn their heads, or act sleep where there is a pregnant woman or elderly person standing on the train. This is some real shit, I am experiencing. Normally, I could take the train anywhere but now it felt impossible. I was so tired from treatment. Inside the train, the air was so thick from 100's of people crammed into a train car like sardines which on average is a 750 square foot space. After a few stops I had enough. I could not take the heat, and the thick funk of the train was unbearable. *(Did I mention that during chemo, some of your other senses heighten, including my sense of smell? Yeah so just visualize you smelling old garbage and funky underarm on a 134-degree day in July in Death Valley, California with no ventilation. Smell my pain?)* Next stop was Borough Hall, I had to

78

remove myself from the train and just in time too, I threw up all over the platform. It was horrible. I found tissue in my bag to wipe my mouth, rinsed it out with the spring water in my bag, and proceeded to the closet bench. *(This is when I knew I was sick, I hate sitting on those benches. Some people that occupy the subway seating is down-right nasty and gross – Yuk)* Not one person asked if I were ok, they just hopped over my vomit to catch their train. I got myself up and walked slowly to the exit, I climbed the stairs at snail pace, by the time I reached the top, it felt as though I ran the NYC marathon. Exhausted. Feeling the cool air on my face and pulled out my phone to get an Uber to go to work. No more trains for me. I started driving into the office 4 days a week, and that was super expensive but worth it. Subsequently after the transportation fiasco, my natural reaction was to anticipate what side effects would come next.

Two days before my third treatment of chemotherapy, I started coming down with a sore throat. I could feel a lump on the right side of my throat. (*PAUSE.... For those of you that reading this, and you have never been a cancer patient, let me tell you how it feels. When a patient experience anything additional after diagnosis that is abnormal their mind immediately goes negative and it freaks them out. It is what it is.*) Is that a lump, oh my goodness; do I now have throat cancer? All of these thoughts are going through my head. I was immediately in the mirror looking at different angles, running my fingers from under my chin to my collar bone. "What the hell?" I said to myself while calling the hospital emergency number at 2am. My neck and head was warm so I checked my temperature and it was 102. I remember the hospital expressing urgency to call if my temperature was 103 or higher. The doctor on call told me to go to emergency room right away. I feel a panic attack kicking in. Should I go? Feeling nervous and overwhelmed. I had a chemo scheduled for the next day, so rationalized with myself and I waited.

When I arrived at the hospital, the receptionist asked to go see the attending physician before my third chemotherapy treatment, unfortunately Dr. Bedoya doctor wasn't in.

"I'm afraid you won't be able to get chemotherapy treatment this week because of the lump in your neck. We hate to interrupt your treatment but I need you to see the endocrinologist for some tests and check to see what's happening here. I'm going to order a biopsy" the attending physician said.

What? All the pain I went through in the previous weeks with the breast biopsy, I would have to go through another one? After I left the doctor's office I went to the reception area and unwillingly made my appointment for the next day. I couldn't fight this, and I needed to take care of myself no matter what physical pain I would have to endure, for the second time. I went to Raquel's house and mentally prepared for the appointment in the morning. I received a call around 6:30pm from the endocrinologist's office. The medical assistant instructed me to take two ibuprofens an hour before the appointment. This would insure less swelling and discomfort from the biopsy.

"Yoooooooooo you up girl, rise and shine?" Raquel's energetic voice carries from an adjacent bedroom. "Let's go, it's 6am" she says. I was up lying flat on my back on a blowup mattress staring at the celling. Raquel offered to drive my car and attend my appointment with me. Which was fine with me besides, I needed moral support to mentally prepare for another painful biopsy. *(Plus I was nervous as shit – real talk)*

Once I arrived at the doctor's office I signed in, because it was so early, I didn't have to wait long and was almost immediately escorted to the back. I felt my life had turned into a series of appointments. I had no control over what was happening. My vitals were taken, and apparently not so good. My temperature sky rocketed to over 103, and I was sent to the emergency room to get a 'few' test run.

Doctors, nurses, physician assistants, probing me, taking blood, asking questions. It had been a long day, we didn't eat, and Raquel had to soon leave as she had been with me since early morning. After several hours, the physician assistant came to talk to me and take my temperature. "The doctor wants to admit you to the hospital. They need to run more tests to figure out what's happening." Looking up the ceiling "Admit me? Really? "How long do I have to stay?" sadly questioning. "Right now, we don't know" as the PA read my vitals. I thought about what I should do since there was no way I could have expected this. Since we drove in my car, Raquel would have to take my car back to her house that afternoon.

"Okay, I'm ready to be admitted. But you know we have to figure this thing out soon. It's almost the end of March and I'm leaving April 3rd for my trip to Italy" I shared with the nurse. With a funny look on her face she said "Well I don't know if you should worry about that right now. Let's get you admitted so we can figure out the problem."

This is the worst, I was thinking to myself, I didn't even have the biopsy yet. I called my job to inform them I would not be coming in the next day. Laying in the ER bed for a few hours, and of course while I had my feet kicked up and watching television finally able to relax, I was tapped on the shoulder. "Excuse me, we are in need of the bed. Do you mind sitting in that chair?" the nurse pointed beyond the ER room curtain to an oversized chair. Of course I looked at her a little perplexed, but obliged. *(Ain't that some bull, when you're not feeling well, and they make sit in a chair in the ER – that was some bull – just venting)* Hours went by, and my oncologist showed up in the ER.

"What is going on?" he asked "How long have you been sitting here?" looking at his watch. "Since mid-morning" I answered and it was now 8pm. "We are going to get you taken care of" he said. Just as I looked up at the clock, Michele and April came busting in the door with dinner. It was almost as if they were straight out of an action movie with their black leather trench coats flying in the wind in slow motion. *(Queue in theme music from Shaft – You damn right!)* I was so glad to see them and the food. At that point I was so hungry and tired, I just wanted to lay down. April and Michele waited with me until I was assigned a room and hear the update of my condition. It was now 10pm and a bed was coming in my direction.

"Ali?" a nurse called.

Finally, "Yes? Over here" I said waving my arms in the air as if I was a ground operator at the airport trafficking in an air plane. "We have a room ready for you." "Do you need assistance getting on the bed?" I smiled and replied no. I was wheeled into a nice spacious quite room as my friends followed close behind. The nurse came in to explain all of the controls on my bed as well as next steps. My friends stayed for a while to make sure I was ok and to check out my room. I turned on the TV and fell fast to sleep.

About thirty minutes later, a white coat came to my room. "Wake up, Nacole, we are going to give you blood thinners."

Barely awake "Blood thinners? For what?"

The doctor looking down at his clip board "To avoid clotting."

"But wouldn't you only worry about clotting if I was bedridden? Which I'm not" slowly sitting up and fixing my head scarf. We went back and forth debating the usage of blood thinners until he saw I was not interested. "Patient, denies usage of blood thinners" he stated to no one in particular, while writing it down on my file. It didn't bother me at all, though I could tell he was uneasy about my decision.

Later on in the late evening the same doctor had chest x-rays requested. What is going on? "If I'm having an issue with my throat, why would I need chest x-rays?" I annoyingly stated. His response was simple, "Oh, well this is a routine for everyone admitted to the hospital." "Huh? Forgive me but that doesn't sound right." It really did sound stupid. "Soooo...let's say I came to the emergency room with a broken toe. You're gonna give me a chest x ray?" I questioned. Not waiting for his answer, I just told him that I was not taking chest x-rays. While I know I should have been focused on other things, all I could think about was how much is this costing me in co-pays. He started writing in his notes. "Patient, denies chest x- rays..." he announced to no one in particular. By this time, it was well into the night and I was quite tired. Finally, the nurses and doctors stopped coming and I was left alone to sleep. *(Just for the record. I ask a lot of questions when I don't understand. And I made decisions that I thought were right for me at the time. Do what is right for you!)*

The next morning, I awakened to about eight doctors looking over me. Everyone came to party, infectious diseases, head/nose/throat, my oncologist, the endocrinologist, and even attending physicians at the hospital. They were all there ready to find out what was happening in my throat. "What's going on?" with one eye open I spoke. "How do you feel?" a voice from the crowd asked, looking at my IV bags. "What's are her vitals?" another white coat questioned. "Has her fever broken yet?" "What's her latest blood pressure reading?" "Do we have her chest x-ray results yet?"

All these questions seem to come all at once from several different people in white coats. Almost gave me the feeling like I was in the middle of a Wall Street trading floor. "Well we are very curious to find out what's happening to you" said the nose and throat doctor. "We need to take a look inside to see what's causing the infection. Can you tilt your head back for me?" He stuck a long white wand up my nose and down my throat. He also checked my mouth and throat. He looked inside with a little flashlight with a camera attached. "I don't see anything out of the ordinary" the doctor stated. Next, the infectious disease doctor had blood drawn and ran tests. And of course while all of this is going on all I can think about was $$$$. By the way, they didn't find anything either. This was getting interesting, but not in a good way.

"I think she should go for her biopsy as soon as possible" someone stated out of the crowd of white coats. Shortly after the white coats left, transport soon came to retrieve me to take me for a biopsy of the throat. Transport was moving me through the hallways with ease, as I watched the faces of others look at me with complexity. Is it my scarf covering my hairless head? I thought to myself, or is it that I look young and they are giving me eyes of lost hope? While I would like to believe it was my scarf, I quickly came to the reality, that their empty stares were that of a death sentence. I had seen that look before. Transport wheeled into the exam room, the ultrasound came first which was quite painful and unexpected. Oh my goodness, the pain of the forceful pressing down on my lump, slooooowly moving back and forth with the probe. I was moved from one room to the other, it was time for the actual biopsy. Having remembered my last biopsy, the anxiety started to set in. The doctor was a petite Asian woman who insured me the biopsy would be painless, "Just a pinch, Nacole" she said. "It won't be too uncomfortable. All you have to do is relax. We are going to go in and draw some fluid out so we can test it." *(Queue the fog machine, rattling chains and creepy music) She* turned her back to me to grab a machete, gun, and chainsaw – LOL nah, just playing, but that's what I felt like when she turned back towards me with that big needle. I started getting very nervous and wanted to leave. This massive, cartoon-sized syringe seemed to be larger than life. I was convinced the doctor was using a meat thermometer needle to extract the fluid. *(Dear qualified medical staff; don't show the patient the needle, just do what you need to do.)*

"That looks like it's going to be painful" I said. "No, no, no" she chuckled with an evil stare bilking one eye rapidly. "It's not going to hurt, it just looks big. You are only going to feel a little pinch." "I don't know about that" I replied skeptically staring at the point of the needle. With hesitation the evil doctor looked at me and said "Well, would you like someone to come in and hold your hand?" "Yes!" I responded with certainty.

They brought in the sonographer that performed my ultrasound to hold my hand. *(Don't you judge me, I needed any distraction from that needle)* She smiled quietly standing on my left side looking over me. After seeing my nervousness, the nurse decided to strike up a conversation with me. After the casual talk, I was instructed to be very still and not to talk anymore. But it was too late, my mind psyched me out of it and I told the endocrinologist the needle was just too big for me.

"Please, wait, wait, waittttttt! I said with my eyes closed tight. It's not that I don't trust you. I just need to know if there is another option." I could feel the heat of what seems to be a laser, I opened my eyes to find the doctor staring at me with one raised eyebrow. *(Oh! she knows how to do that too?)* Staring her in her eye, she saw how serious I was about the syringe. Without comment, she looked at her medical supplies and started digging.

"Okay, now this here is the smallest needle we have, it's for children" she explained. She kept emphasizing how small it was as if I didn't understand. "This needle is for pediatric patients. It's for the babies." "Yep got it" as I smiled. "Perfect. It's fine for me then" I answered. Honestly speaking the 'smaller needle' just looked as big as the other one, but I know I had to get this done.

I turned my head back to the left towards the sonographer. "Nacole, hold very still. I'm going to give you a small needle to numb the area" the doctor stated with a wicked smirk. First, I felt the needle go into my neck. It was happening all over again. My constant moaning soothed me for a moment. "Shhhh, please don't any noise, Nacole. I need you to be perfectly still. Yes?" "No sound please" she started to put the needle in my neck, and started to apply pressure. She then positioned herself almost on top of me to get a better angle. I felt her push down on the elevated area in my throat. The sonographer let go of my hand to stabilize my shoulders to keep them down. Then my legs were being held down followed by my head. I thought I was going to explode from the pain of the needle drawing out fluids.

The pain subsided. Looking at the needle under the light, the doctor says "Mmmm, I don't think I have enough fluid here. I never saw this color before" as she looks at the fluid in the syringe. OMG! What? tears started to fall to the side of my face, it was awful! "Look lady, there is no way I'm letting you do that again. You are going to have to do what it is you need to do with that right there. And if you really, really, really need to go back and draw more fluid, you are going to have to sedate me. That's it" I stressfully stated.

She was half listening but more distracted by the color liquid in the needle as she held it to the light. Did she really have to say that out loud? I didn't want to hear that my neck juice was odd or abnormal from what she'd seen before. I was a nervous wreck; this wasn't helping in any way. "Okay, well that's it. We will send this to the lab and send your cultures in for testing. Your doctor will review the results with you then" she informed me. Finally, over at least for the moment. It was almost as painful as my breast biopsy. Hospital transport came to take me back to my room.

Now approaching my second week without treatment. I had been praying that this lump in my neck was nothing more than an infection. But of course my mind was thinking the worst. Things were not working in my favor. My blood pressure was up and my fever wouldn't break and still feeling horrible. All I could do at this point was eat soft foods and watch movies. My nurse came in the room to check on me.

"Yuh need any ting?" the nurse shouted from the door of my room in her Caribbean accent.

"Yes, I would like to take a shower" looking in the direction of the door. The nurse walking closer to my bed "Well wah yuh need?" "A fresh gown, no two, can you bring me fresh underwear, and some new socks? Oh, and I need soap, a tooth brush, and some lotion." The nurse sucked her teeth. "Dat all? Oh I can see you are going to be one of those patients. I will be back" the nurse said turning away with annoyance. "Where are you from?" I asked before she could leave the room. "Queens" the nurse shouted back. I laughed out loud. "What's so funny?" smiling back at me. Barely being able to hold my laugh in, I said "You don't sound like an around the way girl" "Wah mi sound like?" the stern voice questioned. You sound as if you are from the Islands and not Staten or Long Island either. She laughed. "I'm from Jamaica let mi guh an get yuh tings" as she walked out of the room. She left with a smile on her face and quickly returned with the items that I requested.

"Here tek yuh Gucci gowns, yuh Ralph Lauren socks, an yuh Vicky Secret panties, an here di otha stuff yuh want." All I could do is laugh and say thank you. "Ok den hit di red button pon yuh remote eff yuh need mi." "I will" grinning and waving goodbye.

"Hi, there" a voice from the other side of the room said "Hi" I responded back even though all I wanted to do was get in the shower and sleep. "I'm here because I have two infections, one in each leg" my roommate said, volunteering the information. "Do you want to see? Here come see." I couldn't be rude, so I got up from my bed and pulled the curtain back to properly introduce myself. "You're so young" she stated. I looked like a deer in headlights. Well that was gross, I thought to myself. "Who is your surgeon?" I took a mental note of her response. Won't be going to see that doctor I thought to myself.

Getting ready for my shower. As soon as I put on my fresh robe, my cousin Nino came to visit. As we are sitting there chatting, a doctor entered my room. "Hi, I understand you refused your chest x-ray" she spoke stiffly. "It's not that I refused the chest x-ray, per say, it's just that the doctor told me it was protocol for every patient being admitted to get one, which didn't sound right for me, and I didn't want to be exposed to any unnecessary radiation if I don't have to. And, if he could articulate the purpose or benefit of me having to take the x-ray, I wouldn't have been reluctant to get it." "Oh, well let me say this. We need to see if the infection has impacted any organs further down in your chest. Furthermore, we need to see if the infection is stable or mobile. We also want to make sure your airways are..." She persuasively and effectively ran down the purpose for the test and why it was necessary for me to have. She took all of two minutes to convince me to take the x-ray. "Thanks doc. That's all I really wanted to hear, a thorough explanation of why I am receiving something." X-rays were ordered. *(She shut me up – didn't she? Lol)* The doctor exited the room. My cousin Nino looked at me and said. "That was crazy. You are crazy!" "What was crazy?" I said. "The fact that the doctor is requesting for you to take certain test for your condition and you vehemently said no. You are unconsciously buggin. If they would have told me to hop on one foot, butt naked in the corner with one sock on, facing south I would have."

"Why?" I responded flipping through channels on the TV.

"Because they are the doctors. They are educated on this topic, and they know what they are talking about!" Nino replied "Well, I like to ask questions and I need informative responses so I can make the right decision for me. I am going to let them take the x-ray" "I got to get back to work" he said. "Okay well see ya later hop along" laughing.

I heard a voice calling "Ali?" "Yes." "I am here from transport to take you for an x-ray." The transporter team popped me into a wheelchair and hurried me off to the x-ray room. Along the way, the orderly asked where I was from. Turns out we were from the same neighborhood in Brooklyn. I arrived to radiation after a ten-minute corridor ride, to have tests done. For the rest of the day I did exactly what they asked me to do which included more ultrasound tests, blood work, and being pumped full of antibiotics.

My endocrinologist informed me about the results of the cultures from the biopsy. They were at least able to determine it was indeed an infection but couldn't figure why or how the infection started. She also mentioned that the infection was rare amongst adults. Goodness, what is going on? I had never been admitted to a hospital before, I had been relatively healthy until all of this came about.

I could tell the doctors were intrigued by the process of figuring out what caused this infection. The doctors spent the morning and well into the afternoon probing and analyzing possible solutions. "We haven't found the root cause to this infection but you must continue chemotherapy. We want you to go ahead and make your next treatment appointment as soon as possible." I agreed. I needed my chemotherapy treatment because I was determined to go to Italy.

After four days, I was finally discharged with a list of meds to take. The following Tuesday, I was back in action as I had hoped. My regularly scheduled chemotherapy was in the early afternoon. I continued my 4-5 hour sessions of treatment and I was happy that I was much closer to the friendly skies. That Friday, I boarded a plane with 10 other friends to Italy.

3

Aprile

Life

(*Damn I guess March was a long month too, huh?*) Well the day had finally come. I had one last conversation with my oncologist and sent his office my full itinerary for the next two weeks. Before I left, he already had my next chemo appointment scheduled.

My doctor sent me a list of contacts along my route in case of an emergency. "I will be watching you from here. Go and enjoy your trip. If you have any issues you call me." I exhaled. I was set to board a plane to Italy in a matter of hours. Since I had undergone chemotherapy earlier in the week my energy level was shattered. I also kept pretty private about my illness up until two days before the trip. Actually, out of the 11 of us attending the trip only three people actually knew. I called the organizer of the trip and told her about my medical situation the night before so that she would be informed. It wouldn't have been the best idea for her to check her itinerary and see an added wheelchair service out of the blue I thought. She was glad that I spoke with her just in case anything happened on the trip. I gave all my information to Michele including my doctors, emergency numbers, access to medical records, and medication list, and my travel insurance was secured in case I needed to fly home. I knew I had to take precautions before traveling which the doctor warned me about. After getting everything in order I called Chris to see if he would pick me up from home and take me to April's house.

Chris cleared his voice "What up?" Multi-tasking and sending my itinerary to my niece via email, I asked Chris over speaker phone if he can be my transportation. "You want to come all the way over there and bring you where?"

Looking down at the phone I clarified "To April's house, we are taking her car to the airport."

"When?" he said.

"Thursday."

Hearing construction noise in the background, Chris shouted "I thought your flight was Friday?"

"Yeah, but I would rather already be there instead of rushing on Friday."

"Yeah, what time?"

"I need to be at her house by 8am."

"What? why so early?"

"So I can work from her house on Thursday, unless you want to come get me Thursday night?" "Nah, I will be there Thursday morning at 6am to pick you up, be ready!" With the sound of a truck backing up in the background, he hung up.

Thursday morning arrives and I am packed and ready to go. Zipping up the last of my bags I called Chris to make sure he was on time. "Are you close?"

"Yes, I said I would be there. It's too early for questions."

"Okay, cranky" I said moving my bags close to the front door.

"Look, I will see you when I get there. Bye" as he disconnected the call.

I texted April to let her know I was at her house. Pulling into April's driveway Chris parked the car and helped my inside with all of my bags.

"What's in here a body?" lifting the bags out of the trunk.

"No bodies just those damn wigs. They add extra weight."

Huffing and puffing climbing the front stairs "I can't believe you just said that. You are ridiculous."

"Uh ok." I laughed.

 Kissing me on forehead "Alright gotta go have a safe trip."

 Eyeing him straight in his eyes "Before you go – you know I get back in 12 days, you are picking me up right?

"Yeah, I got you and bring me back a Gucci belt." Looking at him from the top of the stairs "What? What happened to a postcard?" *(People don't ask for simple gifts anymore – damn shame – I digress)* Opening up the car door, he shouted from a distance. "I just got out of my bed drove an hour to your house, drove an hour over here and now I'm going to work – hmmm two Gucci belts!" Amused I yelled "Your extorting a cancer patient?" "Boy oh boy the ish that comes out of your mouth, never mind I will see you when you get back. Have a safe trip." He drove off shaking his head. I closed the door.

Tying up some lose ends, I called ahead to the airline to get wheelchair service at the airport. Later on that evening after April arrived at home, we ate and then we were both up late working on last minute things before our trip. The next morning, Raquel has arrived at April's house and we are on our way to the airport.

Pulling up to the terminal, we saw a few of our travel mates waiting patiently. We greeted everyone and just then, a porter came over with Raquel pushing a wheelchair. There were a few inquisitive eyes but no one said anything. They were trying to figure who the chair was for. "It's for me" raising my hand. Shoot I was bald and tired, wearing a turban, it was cold, and I was doubled tucked away in my down jacket. I didn't waste time feeling shy or embarrassed about the chair. I hopped in and kept it moving.

"Let's get it started" I bellowed with a grin. Everyone followed behind the wheelchair. Not one person asked why I was in a wheelchair. They respected my space which I appreciated. *(Although they were probably talking behind my back – I almost sure of it. Saying things like: why does she need a wheelchair? Why is she wearing that turban? It's cold, but it's not that cold, why is she bundled up like that?)* I wasn't ready to come out and say what the problem was right at that moment, but I can imagine the whispers. We were all going to have fun and enjoy this trip together.

Feeling weak from treatment I pulled myself together and managed to smile and stay pleasant while keeping up with the crew, with a bit of assistance of course.

Wait up a voice yelled from our crew. "April can't get pass security!" Not knowing what the issue was a few of us doubled back "Hey what's going on?" I questioned. Looking annoyed with her hand on her hips, April said with annoyance in her tone, "My passport expires in 3 months, even though we will be back in 2 weeks. So they won't let me get on the flight." *(Sidebar: Most countries will not permit a traveler to enter their country unless the passport is set to expire at least six months after the final day of travel. That means if your passport has less than six months remaining until the expiration date, you will not be traveling)*

Sitting in my wheelchair I asked "So now what?" "This is some bullshit, I can't go, and I have to go to passport office tomorrow, and try to get on a flight in two days? I will catch up with you guys in Venice." How horrible I am thinking to myself. This is the worst. We had been planning this trip for months. "No worries, I will see you guys in a few days" she assured everyone. Leaving April behind, we proceeded to our gate. Taking full advantage of my wheelchair and global entry, we were expedited through long lines at immigration, security check, and even boarding first on the flight. Ahhh the perks.

The flight was comfortable for the most part and I enjoyed a few of the amenities on board even though a few times I felt a bit nausea and fatigue but it was to be expected on our 8-hour flight to Milan. I put on my protected mask, sat back and next stop Milan. *(I was looking crazy but did not care. People were looking at me like – What she got? I kept look back at them with my eyes opened wide, quickly raising my eyebrows up and down trying to telepathically tell them I have cooties. Lol I have to have some fun.)* "Welcome to Milan" a voice echoed through the sound system. When we landed at Malpensa Airport, I sat and waited patiently for a wheelchair and escort. Everyone was debarking, and I was left sitting there. Raquel waited patiently with me taking pics of herself with her selfie stick. After a few minutes, we started to complain "si prega di attendere un momento madam" the flight attendant said "in corso al termine del corridoio." Not knowing how to speak Italian, Raquel and I both looked at each other and started laughing, then waited for the flight attendant to start using hand gestures, we had no idea what she was saying. *(Use Google translate, I did)* Needless to say, I made it off of the plane and was waiting right outside the jet way. By this time, it had been at least 7 whole minutes, but it felt like 4 hours. Finally, in a far distance, I see an airport employee walking briskly towards me – wait for it…. with a black office chair on wheels with no arm rest. Raquel thought this was the funniest thing ever, she could not stop laughing. I was sooooo annoyed. Raquel took out that damn selfie stick and started taking pictures. Without a choice, I took the ride, a nerve racking ride I might add. Oh madam please sit the airport employee said. Frustrated, "I asked for a wheel chair not a chair with wheels, what is this?" Ugh, this is all that we have at the moment with his Italian accent said the English speaking airport employee. I sat on the chair and as he started to push, the swivel chair would not stay straight. We were going up hills and around corners trying to get to baggage claim. I was spinning, and twisting all the way. I was holding on to the sides of the chair with wheels for dear life. I felt like I was the Tilt-A-Whirl ride in Coney Island. What a disaster, I am about to have motion sickness and

Raquel is busy snapping pics and laughing. I am just glad I did not fall out that stupid chair.

Finally arriving to baggage claim, my friends had grabbed our bags while they were waiting for us. Our tour guide had a sign waiting for us as we walked out into the busy sidewalk. She escorted us to our motor coach that would take us directly to our hotel in Milan. "Nacole how are you?" the tour guide marveled. I have known her for years, as I had been on pervious tours with her. "I'm good" I insisted even thought my body was feeling depleted but my spirit was on a natural high. From the smell of the air, the picturesque landscape along the countryside, I was thankful I made it this far. The tour guide was attentive in asking if I needed to stop or use the restroom for any reason and anything that could accommodate my needs. There were only the 11 of us on the huge motor coach which made the experience more unique and private. At this point, my travel mates sort of put two and two together and figured out there was a more serious issue I was dealing with. I could clearly see the emotions in their eyes. Everyone was really compassionate throughout the trip, from offering blankets to slowing down whenever we're walking. It was a blessing to be amongst such good people. We rode along the streets of Milan and chatted about what we would do in the days ahead.

Once we arrived at the hotel, we were in awe of the modern beauty and chicness of the hotel. Our hotel for the next two nights was the UNA Hotel Century, Via Fabio Filzi, 25/B. Since arriving to the hotel, my fatigue was now at an all-time high and the meds for my throat was kicking in. This didn't dampen my spirits though. I already knew that in 1-2 days of the trip, my energy would come back. Being back in Milan was a breath of fresh air. On the other hand, everyone was jetlagged and it was rainy so we checked into our hotel and parted our separate ways for resting. It was a great relief for me to hear that everyone else was also tired and wanted to rest. Thank goodness nothing was planned for the first night.

The next day we were up early and ready to get our day started, even though our bodies were still six hours behind. So what's the plan I heard Raquel say, I turned around to see she was on the phone. I figured she was on the phone with April. "Yeah, that's good. See ya in Venus." Raquel said with excitement. I just assumed I knew what the conversation was about. Oh good I said, everything worked out? Raquel replied "yes." Michele knocks on the door to tell me she is leaving for Rome and will be back the following day. "Rome?"

"Yes honey, me and a few others are going to catch a flight to Rome to see the Pope for Easter Sunday's service." My eyebrow went up with concern, but if you know my cousin you know that she will try and get as much stuff done on her list in one trip if possible. And seeing the Pope on Easter Sunday was on her list. "How are you getting to the airport? Do you have a ticket to get into the

114

Vatican? It's supposed to rain, do you have an umbrella? Without giving her time to answer "Well be safe, call us and let us know that you arrived safe." "I will, I so excited, I am going to see the Pope" Michele said with happiness in her eyes.

Rain, Rain, Rain that didn't stop her. When she arrived in Rome she sat on the ground for hours waiting for the Pope to arrive. And yes, she got a selfie with the Pope riding in his Pope mobile behind her. No he didn't pose for it, but you gotta love the zoom on the iphone, it makes you appear to be closer than what you really were.

"Let's go walk around, I'm hungry" a famished Raquel said. Ha! What else is new? A bunch of us walked over to what looked like a large NYC Penn Station. We looked around and saw an elevator going up to the restaurant level. We crammed on and the unfortunate happened. We got stuck. Yes, we were stuck on the elevator with two foreign exchange students. Why the hell did we get stuck? As one of the ladies was looking up at the capacity sign. "It says maximum 8 people. 1-2-3-4-5-6-7-8" she counted off. "There is only 8 of us on here." "Yes, but I think they mean 8 skinny people like us" one of the foreign exchange students said. *(Please take a minute and re-read the last quote.)* It was almost like a scratched record at a party. It was like an old bar scene when everyone clears the saloon. These two young boys from Mexico in the elevator with 6 'healthy' African American women had no idea what they just said. After a deep breath and a few moments of silence, all we can do was laugh and ring the alarm for help. *(But you know that could have gone from zero to ten really quick – just saying.)* After about 10 minutes help arrived and we were rescued from the elevator. However, in the 10 minutes that we were stuck I think we took about 100 selfies. This was just day 2.

Michele and the others came back from Rome and finally, April caught up with us in Venice 2 days later via 2 planes, a bus, a boat, a gondola, a skate board, a bicycle, and a camel, but

116

she made it in one piece, but I can't say the same for her luggage. All of us are finally here and we are enjoying every moment from Milan to Venice, to Florence, Lake Como, Tuscany, Switzerland, and Rome. We had a fabulous time, Michele randomly serenaded a couple in the Piazza San Marcowe, crashed a wedding, we did endless shopping, we laughed, we had an official Italian style dinner, we did endless shopping, we went to the Vatican, the Colosseum, the Spanish Steps, the Duomo in Milan, museums, a gondola ride, a six course lunch wine tasting in Tuscany, ate amazing food, and did I mention endless shopping. Every time we got back on our motor coach, we would have a full fashion show of all the things we just bought and laugh about it. A trip for the history books, for sure.

Thank your flying Alatia, we hope you had a wonderful flight. You are now arriving Newark International Airport. Welcome back to the US. With mixed emotion our journey was coming to a close. After returning home from an amazing trip in Italy, I was back confronted with the reality of what I was going through. I had a horrible infection in throat and I had chemo scheduled for the next afternoon.

Everyone in the hospital could not wait to hear all about my trip and of course see how I was able to hold up. My oncologist was more than happy to see me with a smile on my face. "All is good? Let's run some test" he said. All of my pre-test came back satisfactory and I was cleared for Chemo. That session was a little hard, as my veins seem to not want to cooperate. The nurse had to stick me a few times before they found a good spot. Finally, the IV is in. I turned the lights off in my room, closed my eyes and fell fast to sleep. Jet lag and chemo are a recipe for a good deep sleep.

Two weeks later I went in for my next session, and as soon and they stuck me with the IV, I could not stop itching. I had an uncontrollable itch that seemed to be under my skin. The inching in my right hand became intolerable. The nurses immediately stopped the IV for fear of an allergic reaction. My hand started to swell. And the dreadful words came out of the attending physician's mouth. "We are sending you to the ER." Damn it! I slammed my head back and closed my eyes and the tears started to fall. I was so upset. What was happening? Why is this happening? It always seems like there is something. I see why people don't want chemo. I see why they give up. This process can become so frustrating and long. They never really tell how long all of this is going to take. I get myself together, and I pulled myself out of my own pity party and gather my belongings.

A few minutes later, I am in the ER waiting to see a doctor. They send me for vitals, and the next thing I know they are sending me to observation. Observation is a holding pattern kind of, not sure they need to admit you, so they just want to watch you for a few hours. Well my few hours turned into 2 days. IV bags hanging with slow drips. I will say the room was pretty cool. I was scheduled to go to a tea party with the girls, but I clearly was not going to make that, so I texted April, Michele, and Raquel to let them know.

The next day after the tea party they came to visit in their pretty dresses. I showed them how cool my room was. All you had to do was wave your hand in front of the glass on my room door and watch it frost over or un-frost. Everything in that room was state of the art. I think Raquel played with the door for about 15 minutes. As a matter of fact, she still talks about it till this day. I was released to go home.

4

May

Lady Sings The Blues

Everyone in the hospital was very nervous because they don't know what happened. I was now known as the girl with the hand. Another biopsy was ordered for my hand, yes another one. My hand had been swollen for days, and they were not sure why. Once again chemo had been put on hold. *(Real talk by this time I was getting tired. I was getting tired of the process, it was taking a toll on me.)* I went to a specialist to take a look at my hand. He took one look, numbed my hand and started to extract fluid. At this point I was feeling angry and exasperated. More fluid samples and more tests.

My doctor talked to me about getting a port. All I could think about was, another thing I have to do. They showed me what the port looked like and then they proceeded to tell me that it was an ambulatory procedure. Another procedure that is all I heard. Tears of frustration fell out of my face. (*You read correctly they fell out of my face, you really don't know the purpose of your eyelashes until you don't have any. My tears had nothing to cling too – it felt weird.*) You will need someone with you that day, and you might be a little tender the first few days, but you should be ok. They will put you in a conscious sleep, the nurse explained. I said no. I did not want another procedure. I did not want them to open me up. My doctor explained calmly why he thought this was necessary. So many decisions I had to make. The stress was breaking me down. After several conversations, my doctor convinced me it was the best option for me.

At that point, it was decided to put a port in for my benefit to minimize infection. I scheduled to appointment and called Chris to see if he could pick me up after the ambulatory procedure and take me to chemo. He agreed.

Although I was dealing with the infection for the entire month, I still have things happening in my everyday life including a business trip that I had to take. I kept being faced with unexplained infections that intimately put chemo on pause, made me nervous, but I could not stop my daily life. Going to the doctor 2 or 3 times a week became my new normal. It didn't matter how tired I was, or if no one could come to the doctor with me, I had to continue on and fight this battle on my own. I refuse to let this illness put me flat on my back. *(It was definitely kicking my ass. I was feeling like Apollo Creed in Rocky)*

In my steps towards recovery there was hope, there was possibility and there were people who are there for me. Throughout the summer I planned to go to tea parties, barbecues, my god-daughters' graduation party and so many other events. I refused to stay in the house. I refused to admit to anyone that this illness was holding me

124

back. Through this process you have to live your life. You can't take anything for granted with your friends and family. You need to make the most of every opportunity to be with the people you love.

.

5

July

Independence Day

What a hot summer, at least for me. Wearing three hats at one time with these wigs. For the life of me I don't know how people do this for fashion. After moisturizing my head, so weird, I put on a wig cap, and then the wig, and then a hat because the wig didn't look natural enough for me. Talk about being hot. I felt like I was in Al Aziziyah, Libya on their hottest day. Every day felt like I was wearing 3 hats, 2 Moncler coats, and sheepskin long johns. And if I not wearing a hat, I put on a scarf. But I made it through until the 31st of July - my last day of my chemo. Holy shit, I am finally, with chemo and things are going to be better now. *(So I thought – keep reading)*

After the machines shut down, I stood tall and proud and took the infamous pic of me on my last day of chemo. I started saying goodbyes, like this was my last day of high school before college. I said so long to my nurse staff that I have come to know and bond with. "Congrats Nacole, you are finally done with chemo. How do you feel?" my nurse said.

"I feel good, about to head out on a weekend get-a-way."

"Of course you are. Well enjoy your trip. See you in 3 weeks" she said.

Stopping in my tracks "Why?" I responded with major concern. She looked at me as like I should have known "Because you still have to get your hormone therapy treatments."

Sitting in the closest seat to me "Yes, I thought that was a pill?"

"At this point you need 14 treatments of the

hormone therapy which is given through IV every three weeks, and then you will probably get a prescription to take a daily pill at home, but your doctors will inform you. You look surprised." Taking a deep breath. So I'm done, but I'm not done? My heart slight sunk. At this point I was feeling like there was no end to the tunnel. My bright light has now once again gone dim. "Ok well see you in 3 weeks." With a disappointed tone "Will the hormone therapy be as long as chemo sessions?" I asked. "No it will be much shorter, maybe a little over an hour." Leaving the room to attend to another patient "Enjoy your trip!" I walked out my chemo room with mixed feelings. I know I had to continue on fighting so if I had to come back in 3 weeks, then that is what it was.

I celebrated that day by taking a local spa trip with Michele, April, and Raquel. We laughed so hard the entire weekend. Michele is always the life of the party, even if she doesn't intend to be. Lunch the next afternoon, was at a restaurant in the spa grounds. Michele ordered some fancy ice tea, and when the tea arrived, she looked down in the glass and saw a small, I mean a minuscule piece of paper floating at the top of her drink. In her dramatic voice *(By the way I don't know why her dramatic voice is an imitation of a valley girl but whatever.)* she calls for the waitress "Ah, excuse me, like, over here" as she waves her finger back and forth. "Like oh my gosh! There is paper in my glass, I mean like I can't drink that! Can you please call the manager?" I am tickled pink, but all I can do is shake my head, but not too hard, don't forget I have a wig on. The manger comes to the table and Michele begins to express her dissatisfaction. "Kind sir, do you see that? As she points to the lint in the glass. That thing like floating in my glass? I went to take a sip, and I like almost choked on the paper." Eyes filled with despair, Michele looked at the waiter. The manager immediately apologizes and agrees to remove the drink from her bill and send her a complementary drink. And the Oscar goes to…. Giggling as soon as the manager left,

130

"What a performance" as I clapped and bowed my head. *(Not too much though, you guys keep forgetting I have wig issues – lol)* Good times. Michele had a victory smile from cheek to cheek. I could not have thanked these ladies more for what they did for me and the sacrifices they made to help me thought this tough time. They brought flowers and balloons to the suite at the hotel and plenty of food.

To celebrate my last chemo with this spa trip was such an amazing gift for me to be with the true friends that I had in my life. There are times when the true colors of our so-called 'friends' come out when we go through difficulties. There are some people who fell along the way as I traveled my road to recovery. There are some people that I have known for 20 or even 30 years who are no longer around. In fact, some of them treated me as though I was already dead and buried.

So I learned a valuable lesson that some people are going to remove themselves from my life and that's okay. Let them fall away and let them stay away because a person who isn't willing to walk through your darkness with you doesn't deserve the opportunity to be with you when you're in your light. *(Let the church say amen –I have to be transparent without the jokes sometimes to let it be heard with no fluff.)*

6

September

Do The Right Thing

In the blink of an eye it was time for my double mastectomy. Unlike some women, I chose chemo before surgery, which in my case I was given the option. After 16 rounds of chemo, and a port inserted, I was ready for the next step. I had a double mastectomy and a whirlwind of pre-surgical procedures and appointments with my breast surgeon and my plastic surgeon. As part of my appointment with my plastic surgeon I had a 'before' surgery photo shoot *(if that wasn't a reality check – I guess I didn't lose as much weight as I thought)*. After the photos I went in the office to wait for Dr. Dave. Dr. Dave was a well-dressed, pleasant looking man. *(Ladies he was fine, tall, in shape, smelled good, and had a bashful smile.)*

Escorting me into the office "Doctor Dave will be in shortly" the nurse confirmed. Hopping up on the exam table and my feet dangling "Thanks!" I said and before I knew it, Dr. Dave walked in the door. Smelling good, and with a pleasant smile. "Nacole, how are you today?" Sitting up straight, and fixing my head scarf "I'm feeling alright" in a tranquil voice "Glad to hear. Well congratulations on completing chemo. I understand you had some issues along the way, but I am glad to see you. Let's discuss the next steps. Did you want implants or **flap reconstruction?**" *(Flap reconstruction is when they use tissue transplanted from another part of your body such as your belly, thigh, or back).* "Going based off what I previously read online, I was hoping to do the flap" I responded. "Let me take a look, please take off your robe" with no hesitation, I took off my robe. As a matter of fact, I think it dropped to the floor before he could finish his sentence. "Well unfortunately it doesn't look like you have enough fat for that" I looked at him partially disappointed. For someone to tell me

135

I don't have enough fat was refreshing on the other hand, that means I will have to opt for implants. "There might be another option" he said. That was music to my ears. "We may be able to do a TUG flap transfer" Not hearing that term before I asked "What is that?"

"The TUG flap uses the gracilis muscle, located in the upper inner thigh to reconstruct your breast" he explained.

"I'm sorry, what does that mean exactly?"

As he traced my inner thigh as he clarified "That means we take the fat from your inner thigh to reconstruct you breast." Trying to understand all that he was telling me, I still was unsure of the process. "How do I know if I qualify for that?"

As the doctor stepped away from the exam table, he sat down on a rolling stool, so he could make an assessment. "Well let's see, please pull your pants down so I can take a look." Ladies, he didn't say nothing but a word. *(Don't judge me, you would have done the same thing)* So I dropped my pants as expeditiously as I could. The doctor started to examine my thighs. As he started to move closer to my vaginal area I started to get a tingling sensation. "Oh my goodness, Dr. Dave – It works – My vajayjay works." He looked at me perplexed" He had no idea of the confirmation he gave me. I was so elated to know that my medication and side effects of chemo has not completely killed the candy box. *(Yippy there is hope for me after all)* "What do you think you want to do?" he asked. So were so many things to think about, I felt like I couldn't answer right then and there. "I am not sure by when do you need an answer?" Rolling the stool backwards and looking at my file he advised me that the two surgeries were very different and take different amounts of time so the sooner the better, as the appropriate amount of time needed to be schedule with the OR. I would soon have to make a decision.

I made a decision to go with the implants. It is the day of surgery, I headed for the hospital early. Taking naked selfies in the mirror to remember my body as I knew it. What am I going to look like? How am I going to feel? I didn't know how to feel. I was numb. Feeling a conflicted, sad, empowered, nervous, and worried all in the same second. I got myself together and ordered an Uber. This feeling is a little surreal. I looked around the house, make sure I had my bags packed, as I would be recouping in Brooklyn. Walking out of my bedroom in the body I had known for 43 years was now coming to an end. Bracing myself.

Arriving early, I thought I could get some last minute things tied up with work. I was on a conference call in the waiting room, when they called me in earlier than I expected. *(Talk about dedicated to the job – gee-wiz.)* It was time, I closed my computer and ended my call. I followed the nurse to the back. I was prepped and given a bed. Shortly after Michele, and Raquel came into my room to wait with me until it was time. I think at least 4 or 5 doctors came in to ask me the same questions over and over. I suppose if I wanted to bail out, that would be the time to do it. A few hours had passed and my surgeon came in for one last check. "Do you know what procedure you are having today? Are you ready?" my surgeon asked in a serious voice. I answered all of her questions. She looked at the nurse and gave her the go ahead. "See you in the operating room" she whispered as walking out of the room.

"Ready? Let's go to the operating room" the nurse said. Looking at the nurse in a confused manner "No, you can walk right?" I replied "Yes, but I don't want to walk through the halls holding my robe tight so my butt is not seen by the world. Besides this is not how they do it on TV. Aren't you suppose to wheel me in?" *(Take one- Quite on the set - Queue the in Young and The Restless theme music, queue the extras running through the OR asking for stats, and the one tear falling from my face as I turn*

139

to see my friends one last time.) Back to reality, with slight attitude in the nurse's voice "You want us to wheel you into the OR?" "Yes, pleaseeeee" Every TV show or movie I have ever seen, the patient never walks into the operating room. Where do they do that? Apparently at my hospital. The foot of bed pushed open the doors of my room and off to the OR I went. I said goodbye to my friends.

(Take Two - Queue the Chariots of Fire theme music. I am going in to win this Olympic race. I am going in there a woman, and I am coming out a woman with a few alterations.) It was like NASA in there, I have never been to NASA, but I like movies I told you. There were screens everywhere, Surgeons, Nurses and other staff were busy talking and preparing for me, busy moving around the OR making sure everything was right. My vitals were posted, my picture *(not a cute one either),* personal information and all. WOW. "Are you comfortable?" Lay back and put your up. We are going to give you the anastasia through your

port. Count from 1 to 10." The nice lady said in a soft voice. I think I counted to 1 before I felt the effects of the anastasia. The only thing I remember is waking up in recovery and telling my God mother that she looked like she was in a broke rap group with her head scarf on. I remember seeing Michele and another friend of mine that came to give me moral support. I was told that I came out of a surgery laughing, joking and telling stories. I guess don't give me morphine unless you want me to talk crazy. I slept the rest of the time until the nurses came in the middle of the night to wake me up and walk me around the hospital as if I requested a tour at 3 in the morning. A few hours later my surgeon had come in and let me know that everything went well and that my lymph nodes were cleared, which is a good thing. A few hours later a nurse came in with discharge papers. In my mind I just had life altering surgery and a major one at that. Ha, from the time I walked into the hospital, until I was released it was less than 23 hours. I was at my God mother's house and resting. It was not as bad as I thought, and my first look in the mirror post-surgery was not as emotional as I thought.

It is overwhelming to look back at it with all the things they did in that short period of time. It also feels different to see the removal of your nipples and your chest sown up. I had done what I had to do for me and my survival. *(Don't worry if you have the procedure you get used to it – boobs are over rated)*

I didn't feel less of a woman. Yes, of course I was sore during my recovery time but I avoided the mirrors for several days. Not that I wasn't satisfied with my surgery, but I could not bear to see the drains hanging off the side with fluid collecting in these little plastic tear shaped containers. My God mother helped me measure the fluid and clear the drains every 12 hours. I was different. I felt different. But I was still a woman. I was still valuable—somebody pretty and somebody that was worth loving. My trio of friends came over a few days after I was home, and brought me some

142

goodies, and of course leafy greens, straight from April's kitchen. I don't think they knew what to expect. When the doorbell rang, I went and opened the door for them. They were happy to see me walking around. I didn't really have a choice. When your God mother is a registered nurse, and she is caring for you, it's just the hospital; waking me up to take medication, and to clean my drains. Make sure you do your exercises she would remind me every morning before she went to work. Over the next few weeks' various friends and family came by the house to say hi and spend time with me.

7

October

Boomerang

I was in the bed recovering, playing with my baby cousin when the hospital name flashed across my phone, which was not unusual. "Hi, is this Nacole?" the voice said on the other end. Continuing to play with the baby I responded "Yes"

"Hi I am calling from the hospital. How are you feeling?"

I assumed it was a wellness check "I'm okay."

With a slight pause "I have the surgeon on the line for you."

"Hi Nacole, its Dr. Madison" I was silent and I put the baby down on the floor with her toys.

"Unfortunately, we found a trace of cancer in one of your lymph nodes when we sent them for further testing. The tears immediately started to fall. "We will have to go back in and remove your lymph nodes. It is untimely your decision, but I highly recommend it." She stated with compassion. Feeling numb and light headed "When?" I asked with a quivering voice. "Next week, I can get you in." the doctor quickly replied. This is not what I expected to hear. It broke my heart to have to go through that process when I was just beginning to think that maybe the worst of it was behind me and now I was starting all over again. I closed my eyes and exhaled as the tears continued to fall.

The following week, I was back in the waiting room waiting…. "Nacole, Nacole Ali" a voice called. I looked up and it was the same lady that had taken me to the back three weeks prior. "Hey how are you? Come on back. Please take off everything and put that robe on as she pointed the robe hanging on the back of the door. Is anyone here with you?" she asked as she was busy taking needles out of the cabinet.

Fixing the robe so my goodies weren't hanging out I said "They will be here later." She saw the look on my face and my overall demeanor "It's going to be fine."

I began to prepare myself mentally for this next surgery. Not ideal but necessary. There were so many questions in my head. I was beginning to scare myself. Too many thoughts, too many what if's. I was beginning to question my decisions. I was getting confused. *(This is probably the worst thing you can do to yourself. After you have thought long and hard and made your decision, unless intuition is saying something different – stick with your decision – don't keep overthinking everything it will drive you crazy – at least that is what happened to me.)* I felt as though it was a giant step backwards. There were a lot of unknowns during this time. I just want to get back to being me. But this next surgery had additional side effects that I was concerned about. How am I going to manage if I am unable to do the simple things like; carrying anything over 5lbs with my left hand, my worries about getting lymphedema.

It was during this time that I felt the real pressure and the real sense of the tragedy of this disease but I was still determined to overcome it. I was driven and a fighter and that I was going to make it. *(By the way when my parents named me Ali I hated it. Now I embrace it for so many different reasons.)* I knew that I had to continue to be pro-active, that I was taking every obstacle as it came along.

When I finally went to the doctor to get a check-up regarding my lymph nodes dissection, they gave me a word that I was cleared to start radiation too. *(Now if you have been following, I have never mentioned radiation, so I was just as surprised as you are now reading this. When does it end? I was thinking the same thing.)* So this was another emotional point in my life. I was like,

148

what? This was wearing thin. Radiation wasn't something that was on the table or something we talked about. I was done, I made it through chemo, then surgeries and we're supposed to move on now. We are supposed to be done, and moving on right?

I had an appointment with Dr. Bedoya and as soon as he walked in he saw it on my face. He saw that this was starting to break me. My eyes expressed the mental beat down. My internal light was dimming. He looked at me with great concern. He said, "You do not look like yourself", and all I could say was "I'm tired."

8

November

Soul Food

More doctor's appointments and more decisions. It was clear that radiation was non-negotiable, it was a must, so right before thanksgiving I checked into Hope Lodge. The lodge was occupied by people with different types of cancer. I was going to be at the lodge the entire holiday season from the 2nd week in November December 31st. Energy or not, I could not stand to be some place for 6 weeks and at least not make it feel a little comfortable. It was just my luck, there was a .99 cents store a few doors down. Even though the weather had started to change, I would get hot easily, so I put on a light jacket and went to pick up a few things. I managed to spend over an hour in that store. *(Almost everything is .99 cents -*

I couldn't help myself – lol). I headed back to my new temporary digs for a restful night. Tomorrow was going to be busy.

The hospital shuttle would come to pick me up every day to take me to my appointments. My first appointment, I went to the hospital early in the morning to be prepped for radiation. I had several appointments in one day, so they could explain to me the process, including giving me 13 small tattoos over the area to be radiated so they can be precise with the machines every time, and a number of other tests were run to ensure I was ready for radiation. And that's also when I met my awesome team of people that were going to take care of me every day for the next 5 weeks.

Going in for radiation daily, 5 days a week for the next 5 weeks was tiresome within itself, plus it was cold and the holiday season. Sometimes my waiting time was almost 2 hours. Why am I here? Why is this still going on? When will it end? Often asking myself on many of days as I sat there and waited for my turn. The longer I sat there the more I began to put things in perspective. There is always someone in a worst situation, but at the time all I could think about was how could this have happened to me?

My radiation team made things a lot easier for me. Every day they would put on some of my favorite rap music from some of my favorite artist to keep me at ease. With the tunes of RUN DMC or Tribe Called Quest, I would close my eyes, listen to the directions my team would give over the loud speaker, while I mentally pictured the music to get my mind off of the procedure. Sometimes counterproductive, as I had to stay still and who can stay still listening to 'Check The Rhyme'. In the famous words of Phife Dawg "Now here's a funky introduction of how nice I am. Tell your mother, tell your father, send a telegram. I'm like an energizer cause, you see, I last long. My crew is never ever wack because we stand strong….." My radiation was an amazing crew. "Are you ready? Take a deep breath, hold it, hold it, and hold. You're doing good, now relax" a voice would say over the loud speaker. Every day I would hear those words. And every day I would go back to my temporary accommodations and relax until the next day.

Thanksgiving has arrived and I am super excited. Family is flying in and my one of my cousins in hosting this year. It was such a pleasure to have a change of scenery from the Hope Lodge. I made sure that I dressed well, but comfortable for the festivities. "You look good" one cousin said when I entered the house. I smiled heading upstairs towards the amazing aroma of good food. When I reached the top of the stairs, there was family from all over the US that had gathered to break bread together and enjoy each other's company. There must have been at least fifty of us in the house, which my cousin anticipated as she constructed an outdoor heated tent for all of us to have one big sit down dinner. It was just amazing. After dinner, my cousin's husband bought his guitar and we all broke out into song, singing and dancing and having such a good time. It was getting late, and time for me to go back to the lodge. We didn't have a curfew, but I had a long drive and my fatigued was starting to kick in. After all I still had radiation in the morning.

9

December

Higher Learning

I was in the heart of New York City and it was Christmas time. The major department store windows were beautiful. Rockefeller Center's Christmas tree was amazing and the light display on the front of Saks Fifth Avenue's building was spectacular. Even though I am born and raised in NYC, this holiday season feel so different. I am so grateful to be able to see and witness another Christmas. The surrounding festivities had given me an idea. When I woke up the next day, I forced myself to walk down 8th avenue to the main post office to read through a collection of Dear Santa letters. The main post office collects all of the Santa letters that children send with their Christmas list. After reading through several letters, I chose seven;

where ten children asked Santa for things of substance and need. (*Trust me – I over looked those letters where the kids staple the Toys R Us pictures, or the letters that the parents write on behalf of their one year old wanting some designer jeans – yeah okay*) Children that I feel like were in need and who were going to be appreciative. I needed to focus on something else other than my health, so I took those seven letters, and started an Operation Santa go-fund me page campaign and raised a thousand dollars during my radiation so that I could give those gifts anonymously. It was such a good feeling. I went to countless stores to get what was on the list from school supplies, to underwear, blankets, clothing, and a giant teddy bear for a toddler. Doing something other than radiation kept my spirit up. (*Don't get me wrong – this wore me out. I love to shop – but now that I can only really use one hand and I get tired easily – this was a struggle but it was worth it*)

By December 22nd, I had fulfilled the

Christmas wishes that filled the letters, and took them to the post office to be mailed out from Santa. I was determined that I was going to have a good Christmas and add joy into somebody else's life. I'm just grateful that I am here to do it.

I thought I was doing very well up until the last 2 days of radiation. That's when my skin started to burn and peel and it was almost equivalent to 3rd degree burns. In my room looking into the mirror, I saw the drastic change in my skin. Oh my goodness, sore to the touch. I covered myself with the prescribed cream then gave me to care for the peeling. Feeling tired and glancing over at the clock, it was now 1 am. Yes, it is now December 31st and today is the day. I looked around the room and began to pack-up. I refused to spend New Year's Eve in this place. While I was grateful, to be at the lodge, and to see another year come in, I wanted to be home in my own bed.

Bright and early I put all of my belongings by the door, and I headed to the hospital. "Are you ready for your last treatment?" one of my radiation team member said. "Of course" I responded "I thought we were going to have a dance off today for my last day" I reminded them.

"Let the party begin" he said. They turned on the music in the room and for about 1 minute we had our dance off. It was the end of another chapter in this process. It was December 31st, and I was ready for my last radiation treatment. I laid back on the table and let them put me into position for the last time. I relaxed to the sounds of rap and closed my eyes. Before I knew it was over. I was 12 hours from the New Year, and my birthday, and I had so much to celebrate. I was able to check out of the lodge and I was able to begin to check in to 2016 — a year of promise, a new year. I could say to myself that I'm finished with the process. I can move on. I haven't lost me and I still have a sense of humor. Walking to my car I remember thinking, if I had waited any longer, this could have been a worst situation and if I had started sooner, it could have been better. *(Queue in Destiny's Child, I'm A Survivor – it's only right and fitting)*

Through the entire season of my illness, I have done all the things I needed to do in order to keep me going. It was difficult at times but not impossible.

Even during my double mastectomy and lymph node dissection surgeries, I still got up and got dressed every day and went to family functions. I spent time with the people who mattered in my life. I have learned the valuable lesson of how important life is and how important it is that we take action. Cancer is only a death sentence if we don't do anything about it. Procrastination is the killer.

I want to stand up for you too and let you know that you don't have to hide yourself. Just be comfortable being who you are. Surround yourself with the things that make you happy. Don't just lay there on your bed every single day. Get up and do things that make you happy. Take action on the things that will keep you going. You can do it. You are a fighter and you will win. This is not just a testament for people battling cancer, but anything that you are going through.

(Enter center stage, bring up the house lights, turn my mic up, and turn the music down.)

This has been an amazing eye opening journey for me and it still continues to be. Honestly, this event has saved my life and it's still saving me. I don't take things for granted anymore. Even something as simple as going to the mailbox is a joy to me now. I love every opportunity I get to spend with my friends and I don't take it for granted. I've learned to live in the moment and to appreciate it. I do everything that I can to live the best life that I can. I eat better now. I follow my heart more. I don't let people and things stress me out like it once did. In a way, what I found through all of this is true freedom. I am learning every day to live my best life and I wrote this book for you because I want to help you live your best life too.
162

I am a Warrior and I am built to last. Are you?

10

The Bonus Chapter
The ish People Say

For those of you that know somebody that has Breast Cancer…

One last chapter, I had to add this.

The ish people say.

It is amazing that people really don't know what to say. It is hard for someone battling with Breast Cancer to muster up the words to acknowledge this disease and say it out loud. And when they are able to utter the words, I have breast cancer, people respond with the dumbest comments. Or shall I say people think they are making 'light' of the situation but the words that unintentionally fall out of their mouths are borderline idiotic. The conversation always starts off with

"Hey, how are you?"

"Things have been better; I was diagnosed with Breast Cancer" "Oh no! my aunt died of that."

Or

"Oh that's too bad, my neighbor's sister's cousin's house keeper died."

Some people dig real deep and reach down and they still say something, just to say something. Okay for the record why in the world would a person say such a thing? Just to make a connection with the health issue? That is the last thing any patient or survivor wants to hear. Some of my other favorites are "Oh well, at least you will get new breast", or "You don't look like you have cancer." I always ask the question, "What does cancer look like?" What are they saying that I don't look like a tumor? Well thank goodness for that.

166

Please do everyone a favor, as your mother always told you; if you don't have anything nice to say, well then just don't say it at all. But if you absolutely fell compelled to say something, say something like "I'm sorry to hear that, or I wish you the best in health and in strength." Because if you say "Oh my goodness, well call me if you need anything" and the patient actually calls you and you don't respond or can't live up to your word – that's so much worst.

People never cease to amaze me. Here is a few examples of why you should be mindful of your words. One time I went on a business trip in between chemo treatments and my colleague, whom I have meant on several different occasions, introduced herself to me. You can only image my face, I was so confused and perplexed.

"I'm Nacole" I said."Welcome to the team." She said. I then stated my name again with inflection in my voice.

"Nacole Ali!"

"Oh my goodness, I didn't recognize you. Did you do something with your hair?" she said.

As a reminder I was in the midst of chemo... So I politely said, "Yes, I don't have any hair." Her face went flush. The moment was priceless. Just for the visual, I wasn't even wearing a wig. I was only wearing a fashionable scarf. My colleague had no idea what to say at that point. She was speechless. I was literally tickled pink. I think there is a word in the sport of football that is quite suitable; FUMBLE. I didn't get upset, there is no reason to. I just give people a look and then purposely make them uncomfortable and hopefully that will make them think about what they said, and with any luck they won't do it again. I crack myself up.

The ish people say. These are true stories. When I returned to my office shortly after my hair started to grow back, a different colleague said to me "I don't know if I like you with short hair. Are you going to get a weave?" Now I can't even begin to tell you how much I wanted to say something, but instead I smiled and said "NO." I guess the moral of those two stories are… be careful! Your workplace can be hazardous to your health.

By the way other breast cancer patients say dumb things as well, so be aware of who you engage in conversation with especially in the doctor's office, and please don't take things personal.

At the half way mark of my treatment, I was at the hospital waiting to have my chemo, and the lady next to me asked "Are you a survivor?"

I looked at her with no eyebrows and eyelashes and said, "I'm working on it."

"Oh, are you on Taxol? she said. After saying yes, she then proceeded to tell me every bad thing that happened to her while she was on the same drug. It got to the point that I looked at my cell phone and took a call that didn't exist and excused myself. I could not believe that she would be so negative. But then again so many people had made off the wall comments, but I didn't expect it from other patients. And I will admit there has been a time or two, I have unintentionally made a comment to a fellow patient, and oh boy did I put my foot in my mouth.

I was in the waiting room waiting on my chemo treatment, and there was another lady siting talking to her family about how she is going to lose her hair. Soooooo I butted in and said "Don't worry, it's going to grow back" and she looked at me with a 'mind your business smile' and politely responded. "It's not going to grow back, my cancer has metastasized and I will be on chemo for the rest of my life." So after I picked my face up off the floor, I tried to think quickly and said "Well I am sorry to hear that, but try to focus on taking care of yourself, hair is over rated, and then I showed her my head" and she smiled. But boy did I learn my lesson.

Every time I think about the 100's of comments people have made, all I can do is laugh. At times I have had some fun with it, to show people that they should think about the words that come out of their mouth. When people make dumb comments like this, remember these responses.

(Wait queue the theme music for the Benny Hill show)

"What size are breast are you getting?" Triple Z

"Can I touch your head?" No, it's contagious.

"Lucky you, at least you will lose weight." Yes but only in my pinky toe.

"Your skin looks good" Thanks, there is a special chemo soap I use.

"You don't look like you have cancer" Oh do you have a picture of cancer so I see what it looks like?

"At least you get time off of work" I know right, Cancer over work any day.

"Can I touch em?" No they are not sewn on right

"You should wear makeup, so other people around you would feel better" I am, it's called Kiss My A$$.

"How do you know if your treatment is working?" Cause I'm not dead.

"Your hair looks so soft and nice, what type of products do you use?" I use Chemo shampoo and therapy conditioner.

"I saw a movie where the woman dies of breast cancer, did you see it?" No, I didn't what's the name of it, I will watch it right before surgery.

"My colleague had his toe nail removed because of cancer, do you think it would be helpful to speak to him?" Yes of course, because toe nail removal and double mastectomy is like the same surgery.

"I heard if you just eat organically you don't need chemo. Why are you getting chemo?" No reason, I just decided to live.

This journey is what you make it. Like I say on my Pink Notes blog on my website Nacoleali.com, don't read too much, don't assume too much and I can't not stress this enough, do not ask for too many opinions, or get too many people involved in your decision making process. Don't confuse yourself. Or, if you are a survivor be mindful of the feelings new patients are going through; they are seeking the guidance that you wish you had.

Don't forget everyone is different, every diagnosis is different, so take things out of the conversation that apply to you and then consult your doctor.

For more tips please visit follow my blog Pink Notes on www.NacoleAli.com

Made in the USA
Middletown, DE
24 September 2019